THE
3-SEASON
DIET

Also by Dr. John Douillard

Body, Mind and Sport

THE
3-SEASON
DIET

Eat the Way Nature Intended:
Lose Weight
Beat Food Cravings
Get Fit

JOHN DOUILLARD

 THREE RIVERS PRESS • NEW YORK

To My Readers

Do not attempt a weight-reduction or exercise program unless and until you have had a thorough examination and consultation with your physician. As with any diet or exercise program, if at any time during the program you experience any discomfort or serious symptoms consult your physician immediately. If you experience any pain or discomfort during any of the recommended exercises stop immediately and consult your physician.

Copyright © 2000 by **John Douillard**

Published by Three Rivers Press, New York, New York.
Member of the Crown Publishing Group.

Random House, Inc. New York, Toronto, London, Sydney, Auckland
www.randomhouse.com

THREE RIVERS PRESS is a registered trademark and the Three Rivers Press colophon is a trademark of Random House, Inc.

Originally published in hardcover by Harmony Books in 2000.

Printed in the United States of America

Library of Congress Cataloging-in-Publication Data
Douillard, John.
    The 3-season diet : eat the way nature intended to lose weight, beat food cravings, and get fit / John Douillard.—1st ed.
    1. Reducing diets. 2. Biological rhythms. 3. Appetite. I. Title: Three-season diet. II. Title.
    RM222.2.D677   2000
    613.2'5—dc21   99-058302

ISBN 0-609-80543-6

20 19 18 17 16 15

First Paperback Edition

Acknowledgments

THANK YOU TO ALL my patients and students over the years who have proven time and again to be my best teachers. To my wife, Ginger, and my five children for the constant reminders that family life and love are the most important things. To my biggest fans, my Mom and Dad and my sister, Debbie, and her husband Doug, I feel your love and support everyday.

To Peter Occhiogrosso who had the genius to take my voice and vision and turn it into these printed pages. To my editor, Peter Guzzardi, Tina Constable, and everyone else at Harmony Books, thank you all for making this project so enjoyable. To my agent, Murriel Nellis, thank you for finding Peter Occhiogrosso and for all of your support. To Nancy Azeez, thank you for so generously offering to do such a great job on the illustrations on a moments' notice.

Above all, I would like to thank God for . . . everything!

Contents

Preface

OVER MILLIONS OF YEARS of human evolution, nature has figured out how to feed us with astonishing accuracy. The more deeply you study the 3-Season Diet, the more logical and compelling you will find its wisdom. And the proof is in the craving: When you practice this diet, you will crave exactly what nature is about to harvest. You will not experience any struggle or strain, only a growing appreciation of how nature has designed the best diet for balancing weight, mood, and energy for everyone living anywhere on the earth.

In the late 1980s, I went to India to study their natural system of medicine, called Ayurveda. That ancient Sanskrit word means literally "the science of life," an in-depth study of nature itself. To the masters who described Ayurveda in the ancient Vedic texts, perfect health was a reflection of a life attuned to the changing cycles of nature and with all plant and animal life. They saw that these cycles, from annual growing seasons to daily rhythms, were connected to the rhythms of the cosmos and influenced every aspect of nature. Because Ayurveda was derived from natural rhythms, its research and proving ground was found in the expression of nature itself. The 3-Season Diet that I am presenting here is based on the Ayurvedic nutritional map, but with some important differences.

After my postgraduate training in Ayurvedic medicine in India concluded in 1989, I returned to the States and started teaching Ayurveda to doctors and lay people. During my years of teaching, I realized that the original Ayurvedic diets, which work for India, don't always fit well in our culture. So I began to apply the concepts and rules I had learned in India to the pace of life and the foods that are available here in the West. I have spent the last 10 years translating Ayurvedic concepts into the American way of life, including diet, exercise, eating habits, and stress-prevention techniques—all of which are included in this book. The deeper I delved into nature and its growing seasons and harvests, the more respect I had for nature's wisdom. I discovered that the principles of Ayurveda provide a universal body of knowledge that applies to every culture and each individual in all parts of the world. Although I would not call this an Ayurvedic book, the principles from which the 3-Season Diet is derived have been proven over more than 5,000 years. In fact, I like to think of the 3-Season Diet as an updated version of the original American Diet. It is based on the same logic farmers have been using to feed us since the very first harvest.

You Can Eat It All

PART I

CHAPTER 1

The Diet Dilemma and the Eye of the Hurricane

OR SOME TIME NOW, the people of the United States have been overweight in record numbers, and the situation is worsening with each decade. In the last 10 years alone, the rate of obesity in this country has increased from one in eight people to one in *five!* According to the most recent government survey,* 55 percent of the adult population—97 million people—is overweight or obese (weighing more than 30 percent over their ideal body weight). As a result, the same survey states, Americans are spending $100 billion a year fighting weight gain and obesity. More ominous still, the Centers for Disease Control reports that 22 percent of American *children* are obese, twice the level of the mid-1980s.

This epidemic of weight gain has led to a seemingly endless wave of miracle diets, each offering the panacea of weight loss with only a minimal adjustment of one's eating habits, and each promising permanent results. Yet a 1992 study conducted by the National Institutes of Health found that an astonishing 99 percent of all people who did go on diets regained every pound they had lost within three to five years after completing the diet! I don't believe that we are simply weak and lacking in

---

Source: Federal Obesity Clinical Guidelines released in June 1998 by the National Heart Lung and Blood Institute in cooperation with the National Institute of Diabetes, Digestive and Kidney Disease.

sufficient willpower to stay with these diets. On the contrary, I think that most dieters perform heroic feats of deprivation that are not really necessary to begin with.

In the years I've spent working with people who had problems reducing or maintaining their weight, however, many of my clients have come in complaining of weight problems, only to reveal on closer examination that they have difficulty handling stress, or finding enough energy to balance the demands of working and raising a family. In some cases this potent combination has led to chronic exhaustion, fatigue, anxiety, and depression, which they often have to treat with antidepressant drugs. Conversely, patients coming to see me for help with depression and fatigue have very often reported difficulty controlling their eating habits and their weight. It didn't take me long to realize that the connection between overeating, overweight, fatigue, and depression also extended to poor diet and lack of proper exercise. And the clincher is that the weight-loss programs so many of my patients had embraced before coming to see me only made their condition worse. This dilemma is summed up rather succinctly in the recent case history of a patient I will call Jason.

JASON'S STORY

When Jason came to see me, he was pretty much at the end of his rope. He had heard me on the radio show I co-host describing how I had treated one of my patients suffering from weight gain and depression with a totally new approach to diet and exercise. Although Jason had no idea at the time that the two symptoms were related, he came to me because he, too, suffered from a numbing combination of manic bipolar depression and out-of-control weight gain. Several years ago he had weighed 150 pounds, but he was now at 220 and climbing, including a 20-pound gain in the last 4 months. Jason had been on numerous diets with little success, and after 6 months of his latest regimen—a high-protein diet that he had heard about on TV—he found himself completely unable to control his eating. His wife, Susan, who accompanied him, said that not only had she never seen Jason binge on food so much in his life, she had also never seen him so depressed. He had been taking one antidepressant after another prescribed by his psychiatrist; each one worked for a while until he complained of the side effects. In the last month, for instance, his hands, feet, ankles, and other parts of his body had started to swell up. His medical doctor had run a full gamut of tests and X rays but found nothing wrong.

While interviewing Jason, I learned that initially he had lost a few pounds with the high-protein diet, but then inexplicably had started gaining again. I asked him if he was craving anything and he replied that, as a matter of fact, he craved *everything*. "I'm starving all the time!" he said with visible anguish. When I asked if he could be more specific, his wife jumped in and said that she had noticed he was craving carbs and sugars like crazy. "I would catch him eating pancakes off the kids' plates at breakfast," she said, "and he would still be hungry!" For the first time in his life, Jason's appetite was totally beyond his ability to control.

I explored Jason's depression further in an attempt to identify the underlying cause. He was a busy executive who was shouldering lots of responsibility; he had to remember hundreds of details and delegate jobs to numerous people all day long. I told him that a large part of his problem stemmed from stress, which we now know is linked to 80 percent of all disease, and that his body was responding to every aspect of his life as a constant emergency. "You got that right," he said.

Then I explained our plan. "We have to teach your body how to handle the stress in your life calmly, without the constant sense of emergency."

Perking up, he asked, "Is that possible?"

I responded with my favorite analogy. "Look at a hurricane," I said. "The eye of the storm is calm and almost motionless, yet the bigger the eye, the more powerful the winds that surround it. You have lost the eye of your hurricane. We have to restore to your nervous system a calm that will become the central hub of everything you do."

To begin with, I addressed Jason's daily eating habits. Once again, Susan jumped in and said that he rarely ate breakfast, just coffee, and was always too busy for lunch, with the result that he was generally starving by mid-afternoon, and by six o'clock was totally wiped out physically and emotionally. All afternoon he would inhale soda, coffee, candy bars, and corn chips to keep him going, and he had been doing this for 20 years.

I told Jason that our next goal was to get him to make it through each day without craving anything. "If you have a craving," I said, "it means that your body needs something so badly that it sends up an emergency flare, which triggers the release of stress-fighting hormones and free radicals—potentially damaging molecules that are the primary cause of disease and aging. That's all right in a real emergency, but if you do that day in and day out for 20 years, you're flirting with disaster."

During our session, I gave Jason a quick survey of the events that had led him to his present state of near-despair. Restricting the kinds of foods he could eat on the diets he'd been following tended to cause cravings, usually for sugars in various forms, to which he eventually gave in by bingeing. That fluctuation between restriction and bingeing creates peaks and valleys in the blood sugar levels that control our feelings of energy or depletion. Over time, fluctuating energy levels lead to physiological exhaustion, deep-seated chronic fatigue, and finally depression. Overweight by itself is only part of the problem—a symptom, but a very disturbing one. You may be able to make it go away for a while, but if you don't address its underlying causes, it will return with a vengeance— as Jason was discovering firsthand.

Finally, I explained that I wanted to replace Jason's high-protein diet with a weight-balancing plan that I had perfected over years of working with clients with his very problems. This plan, I told him, would reset his body's ability to metabolize fat as fuel—something it had lost because of stress generated over 20 years of disastrous eating habits and deprivation diets. "As long as your body thinks life is an emergency," I informed him, "you will crave emergency fuel in the form of carbohydrates and sugar, and you will mistakenly blame them for your weight gain. The real reason is that in this emergency, the body thinks it will never get enough to eat again, so it stores emergency sugars as fat for back-up fuel. That's why you keep gaining weight even when you go on diets."

Jason nodded his head in agreement, but his eyes expressed confusion. "I don't get it," he said. "What about all the research? I thought these diets were supposed to be scientifically proven!"

I sympathized with Jason, all the more because I knew he wasn't alone. Recently, for example, another patient of mine told me that she had read the best seller *Potatoes Not Prozac* and decided that she was not eating enough complex carbohydrates to balance her moods, as recommended by the author. Like Jason, Cynthia had been suffering from a troublesome combination of weight gain, mood swings, fatigue, and incipient depression. Impressed by the scientific studies cited in the book, she began eating lots of potatoes. Then she picked up the best-selling diet book *Sugar Busters!* and found that potatoes have the highest "glycemic index" of any vegetable (meaning that they contain more sugar and place a higher level of stress on the pancreas); therefore potatoes are to be strictly avoided! Both books claim that the diets they promote will result in improved general health, higher energy, weight loss, and balanced blood sugar levels. "The most confusing part is that both books are backed up by good research and science," Cynthia had lamented. "Who do I believe?"

The fact is that the authors of both those books are right to some extent, as we will soon see. I have great respect for scientific research when it is done properly; the problem is that we have such an abundance of research today that by citing selectively, authors can back up just about any claim that suits their dietary agenda. Furthermore, for every scientific study that supports a high-protein diet with irrefutable results, I could find another equally unimpeachable study that will show such a diet is potentially harmful. The same is largely true for each diet to appear over the past fifty years or so. Why is it so difficult for us to agree on a single diet that will work for most humans?

The answer is so simple that I am amazed by how many contradictory diets have been able to proliferate for so long, all missing the point. We don't find much discussion of diets in the natural world. Animals know nothing about proteins, carbohydrates, fats, or calories, yet they are just about the only beings left on the planet with perfect nutrition. Animals have lived by the same program of food consumption for millennia, just as our ancestors did. Yet during the last century, despite our supposedly superior knowledge of science and our grasp of technology, we have been taking a very unsettling roller-coaster ride from one ineffectual diet to the next. The reason for this unacceptable state of flux is that each new diet has merely attempted to solve the problems created by the previous diet without ever addressing the root cause of those problems. Unfortunately, as I will show, what we get from these diets is symptomatic relief that does little or nothing to identify or resolve the underlying issues.

After studying nutrition, fitness, and weight management and working with thousands of patients over the past 19 years, I have come to some simple but startling conclusions. The fad diets with which we as a nation have suffered for decades can be reduced to three essential types: low-fat/low-calorie diets, high-carbohydrate diets, and high-protein diets. Not only can proponents of each of these kinds of diets cite the latest scientific research proving that theirs is the only diet you will ever need, they can also support claims that the other two kinds of diets are inappropriate and even harmful.

Pick up a book promoting the Pritikin, Dean Ornish, Fit for Life, or any other low-fat, low-cholesterol, or high-carbohydrate diet and you will find competent scientific studies establishing beyond the shadow of a doubt that a high-protein diet causes weight gain while putting the body at a greater risk of certain kinds of disease, including cancer. You will also learn that the human body was designed to eat fruits and vegetables, not to devour meat, fish, and poultry. Then pick up a high-protein diet book such as *Dr. Atkins' Diet Revolution* or the Eadeses' Protein Power Diet book and you will be confronted by equally impressive research contending that humans have been eating meat since we first evolved and that our downfall was caused by—you guessed it—the development of agriculture and the increased availability of grains and other complex carbohydrates. This second group of books claims that if you eat only protein—all you want, in fact, including heavy cream, mayonnaise, and lots of red meat—you will lose weight and feel more energetic than ever before.

So I'm not surprised when patients walk into my office totally confused about their diet because they have just come from the bookstore and don't know which well-researched, doctor-approved, best-selling diet to believe. The only research lab that I've found to be proven consistent over a long period of time, however, is nature itself, which has been feeding humanity for thousands of years without the least confusion. Nature's blueprint for our nutrition is an annual cycle, not a daily one. In nature there is no such thing as an RDA (Recommended Daily Allowance), because it is a flat-out impossibility to meet all of your nutritional needs in one day or even a few weeks; it takes a year to meet all those needs. As the seasons blend into one another, we change the clothing we wear, the outdoor activities in which we engage, even the way we set our clocks. But how much thought do we ever give to changing the kinds of foods we eat?

THE 3-SEASON DIET

The question raised by diet gurus and their conflicting nutritional research has a surprise answer. They are *all* right—but only *in part*. Each of these diets works—but for *just about 4 months of the year*. Nature actually designed each of these diets into our lives on a cyclical, seasonal basis, never intending any single diet to get us through the entire year. When people first hear of my 3-Season Diet, they usually ask what happened to the fourth season. The seasons I'm referring to are three growing seasons and harvests that have their conceptual roots in the oldest medicinal traditions on earth. According to the 5,000-year-old system of health and medicine known in India as Ayurveda, the year is more properly divided into six seasons that can ultimately be reduced to three primary growing seasons and three harvests. (Chinese medicine, incidentally, divides the year into *five* seasons, which is most likely owing to climate differences).

In nature, one of the four traditional seasons is always a dormant or resting season, most commonly winter. If you lived on a farm, you would naturally follow a 3-season diet, eating and craving the foods harvested with each of the three *growing* seasons. Now, so you are not restricted to eating only locally grown foods in season, foods from around the world are classified into one of the three harvests. You can eat it all—just wait until it is in season.

The first harvest comes in spring and consists mainly of roots, sprouts, and bitter greens that burst from the ground aided by spring rains and melting winter snow. Summer provides a much more plentiful and longer-lasting harvest of fruits and vegetables that are picked continually during its extended growing season. Finally comes the fall harvest that precedes winter, gathering the last growths of vegetation along with the nuts and grains that will see us through the long winter months. This is when the grapes are harvested and crushed to make wine, when people traditionally put up preserves and gather hay into barns. I refer to this season as winter because although the foods are harvested in fall, they serve us all through the long, cold winter months.

These three harvest seasons translate easily into the three major diets as I described them: low-fat/low-calorie in spring, high-carb in summer, and high-protein in winter. In nature, both animals and humans have always gotten most of their protein and fat for the year in the winter months—just think of squirrels and nuts—and have gotten rid of the excess protein and fat in the spring with a naturally occurring low-fat diet of spring greens and sprouts. During the summer, when the days are longer and the body needs more energy, nature provides us with an abundance of high-carbohydrate fruits and vegetables for boundless vigor and vitality. Based on this observation, one could say (although not exactly) that the Dr. Atkins Diet, or Michael and Mary Dan Eades's Protein Power Diet, both of which recommend getting 80 percent of your calories from *protein,* are somewhat good *winter* diets. Dean Ornish, Jenny Craig, and Weight Watchers—all *low-fat, low-cholesterol* regimens—work well in *spring.* Pritikin, Eat to Win, Potatoes Not Prozac, Fit for Life, and various vegetarian diets that stress getting 70 to 80 percent of your calories from complex *carbohydrates,* are excellent in the summer.

In one sense, then, all these diets are right—but not for the rest of your life! They each work best for about 4 months of the year, although as promulgated they are also a bit more restrictive than might occur naturally. The problem with trying to follow any one of them all year round is that it leaves out two-thirds of nature's requirements—or what I sometimes call your Recommended Annual Allowance. The imbalance created by such a restrictive diet will eventually manifest as a craving for what that diet denies you, whether it's carbohydrates, protein, fats, or sweets. Humanity has survived all this time without counting calories or carbohydrate and fat grams—and without our current epidemic of obesity and heart disease. When we had an agricultural society, people ate much more naturally than we do today, consuming different kinds of foods as they became available in different seasons, balancing their intake of protein, carbohydrates, fats, and sugars. They might have gained a little weight in the winter—just as bears do as they go into hibernation and their metabolism slows—only to burn it off in spring and summer as our metabolism picks up along with the workload and day-light hours. It's no wonder that people cannot stay on fad diets for long. In an attempt to manipulate or trick the body into burning fat, those diets restrict the foods our bodies have long been conditioned to eat at certain times of the year. Whenever you restrict certain foods from the diet for long periods, the body will naturally begin to crave what it is not getting, and that begins the cycle of binge eating, weight gain, guilt, and depression, followed by yet another heroic attempt to stick to a new restrictive diet. Protein, carbohydrates, fats, and sugars are all essential to total health, and in much more balanced ratios than most diets would have us believe. To attempt to eliminate or severely restrict any of these groups will not only fail to bring about lasting weight loss, but will also create health problems down the road.

These highly restrictive diets also complicate the matter of eating, which should be as natural as breathing, and a source of pleasure and contentment. How contented can you feel when you're doing long division to decide what percentage of the calories in a piece of bread comes from fat? Yet the prevailing attitude embraced by many diets seems to be, "If it feels easy, something is probably wrong." I have my own golden rule that I will ask you to follow as you read this book and practice my suggestions: "If you don't like something, don't do it!" The reason is simple: If you are doing something you don't like, you probably will not stick with it. For the past twenty years, for example, 80 percent of Americans have not exercised regularly, and that figure has held constant, despite all the articles about exercise in health magazines and the rising number of fitness centers nationwide. People don't stick with exercise because they don't like it. They often say that they would do it if

QUICK START

To GET STARTED right away, turn to the 3-Season Grocery List on page 109 and simply shop from the spring list in spring, the winter list in winter, and the summer list in summer. Without even noticing that you are making dietary changes, you will be eating with the seasons and craving foods that are coming into season.

they had time, but as you know, if you really like something you'll find time for it. (If you really like ice cream, you don't have trouble making time in your busy schedule for a dish of Ben & Jerry's!) As the old Chinese master Lao-tzu said thousands of years ago, the harder you try, the less success you will have.

EATING MEDITERRANEAN STYLE

Before you get the idea that I just don't like popular diets, let me say that there is one diet that deserves the attention it has received in recent years. A study conducted a generation ago by Dr. Ancel Keys and colleagues at the University of Minnesota examined the relationship between diet and heart disease rates in seven countries and found that people who lived near the Mediterranean Sea suffered vastly lower rates of heart attack and coronary death than those who lived in the United States and other Western industrialized nations. The researchers discovered that their Mediterranean subjects consumed dietary fat that was mainly derived from vegetables, as opposed to the highly saturated animal fats from meat and dairy products consumed by the subjects from other industrialized countries. The so-called Mediterranean Diet was found by subsequent researchers not only to ward off the risk of heart disease but also possibly to help prevent a number of common cancers. But the best part of the diet was that it was so easy to follow and the food was so enjoyable that most people who were put on it tended to stay on the regimen. It seems that enjoying what you eat is the first step to good health—proving my golden rule!

What researchers did not fully understand about the Mediterranean Diet, as they tried to pigeonhole it into some version of counting fat, carbs, and proteins, is that the people in those regions just ate what was seasonally available. What they ate was closely connected to the produce of local farmers and to nature's harvests, combining generous servings of fruits, vegetables, grains, legumes, and nuts with moderate portions of fish and only occasional red meat or dairy. They also took time and relaxed during meals rather than eating on the run or while driving. It's such a reasonably balanced diet that for many people it would be far preferable to the Standard American Diet (or SAD). But by altering the ingredients somewhat from season to season, and by broadening and fine-tuning the range of foods available, especially fruits and vegetables, we can easily improve on the basic strengths of this diet with one that will leave you craving exactly what you need, as each season sets you up to crave the harvest of the next one.

Unlike so many fad diets, the Mediterranean way of eating is not based on an arbitrary manipulation of scientific data, but on traditional agricultural wisdom. Like the so-called French Paradox—the fact that people in France and certain other countries eat a diet rich in fats, yet have less than half the rate of heart disease and obesity than we do—the Mediterranean Diet stresses simplicity and enjoyment without excess.

KNOW YOUR BODY TYPE

I told my overweight and depressed patient Jason that the next step in bringing him back into balance was to read his owner's manual. Whether you drive a Volkswagen, a pickup truck, or a Porsche, you have to know that vehicle's specific requirements to keep it in good running order. If you do not know whether you are closer to a sports car or a family sedan in basic metabolic body type, you're going to run into trouble sooner or later. Your basic body type is derived to a large extent from your ethnic heritage, as we will see when I discuss constitution in more detail in chapter 7. If your ancestors hail from the Mediterranean region, Scandinavia, Asia, or Africa, you are likely to share body type qualities indigenous to those areas. Many recent diets base *everything* you eat on your individual body type or blood type (which is itself related to ethnic roots as well). These diets certainly have merit, and I do believe that your individual type needs to be taken into account. But individuality should be an overlay on what nature harvests, a way to fine-tune your basic diet to to the seasons and your ethnic background rather than dictating the diet itself.

Everyone is different, but just as I believe that all diets can be reduced to three essential varieties based on the three harvest seasons, so all body types can also be reduced to at least some combination of three basic types that correlate to the same three seasons. Some people are cold all year long, and are considered "winter" body types. Others are warm the year round, and so are said to have a "summer" body type. And still others retain water all year, giving them a "spring" body type. Based on which body type you resemble most closely, you can fine-tune and individualize my 3-Season Diet to make it even more appropriate for you. In chapter 7, I will show you how to identify your predominant body type or types, and will help you use this information to mold the basic 3-Season Diet for your specific needs.

I explained to Jason that his particular type had a lot of fire and heat. In the summer he would get overheated and stressed more easily than in spring or winter, and when he overheated he would get angry. Because he had more of a summer constitution, he would need to eat cooling foods from the summer grocery list, which I provided for him, more strictly during those hot summer months to avoid overheating. Like Jason, most of us need to emphasize one or two of the seasons that predominate in our body type. The point is that we all must eat with the seasons, but once you know which seasons you favor, you can adjust your diet to suit your individuality. For an in-depth discussion of body types, turn to page 133.

THE SURVIVAL RESPONSE

Perhaps the most serious problem with highly restrictive or "starvation" diets is that the moment the body senses that it is being starved, it goes into what is known as "emergency" or "survival" mode. When the body perceives an emergency—because it is being starved of either fats, protein, or carbohydrates, or is under extreme stress of any kind—it responds in precisely the opposite way from what we want. Under stress the body produces a degenerative stress-fighting hormone called cortisol, which triggers the body to dump stored sugar from the liver and muscles into the bloodstream. Insulin levels rise to get the blood into the cells to make that emergency energy available. High amounts of insulin inhibit the burning of fat for energy and store available fat for later use. The body responds by craving more "emergency" fuel that is high in sugar and carbohydrates. In a genuine emergency—a life or death situation—the body needs quick energy to fight or flee.

Unfortunately, if the body is responding not to a real life-or-death emergency, such as the sudden appearance of a predator or human enemy or some natural catastrophe, but to the stress of a starvation diet, it responds in much the same way. The emergency fuel the body craves, in the form of chips, chocolate, cola drinks, cookies, and breads, provides temporary, symptomatic relief, but ultimately leads to low blood sugar, lower energy levels, and another craving. The survival mentality generates overeating, overweight, and the thousand ills that too much flesh is heir to.

The same survival mentality, when applied to exercise, can have equally counterproductive results. No diet plan, however balanced, can work to perfection without some consideration of exercise. Unfortunately, exercise has become one more source of stress in our lives, presented in such a punishing way that it either harms the body or is so unenjoyable that most people eventually give up regular exercise altogether rather than prolong the agony. Clients who come to me believe that exercise has to hurt. They have accepted the prevailing wisdom of "no pain, no gain," which says that we have to break ourselves down physically to build ourselves up and burn fat. Once again, the facts are just the contrary. The more intensely you exercise, the more carbohydrates and sugar you burn for energy; the less intense the exertion, the more fat is metabolized as energy. Workout intensity and fat burning are inversely proportional to each other (see Figure 1, page 192) because fat is the body's nonemergency fuel and sugar is used primarily in survival situations. No wonder people get frustrated. Because conventional exercise also builds muscle and stores fat, both of which are heavy, after weeks of sweat and tears at the gym devoted to working off the pounds you can actually *add* weight!

When people exercise strenuously, they usually find themselves huffing and puffing in the name of weight loss or fitness. Unfortunately, this gasping for air is perceived by the body no differently than if you had been confronted by a bear in the woods, a tornado, or a maniac with an assault rifle. It will trigger degenerative, stress-fighting hormones and the release of damaging free radicals. In emergencies, your adrenaline flows and your heart races for good reason, and you don't care if you sustain minor injuries, because your survival is at stake and anything goes. But if you lived that way every day, you would soon have trouble maintaining both your physical and mental health—like soldiers who suffer post-traumatic stress after years of combat. Yet this is what we do to ourselves, albeit less intensely, when we stress our bodies with strenuous exercise and the wrong food. But not to exercise at all can also be debilitating, so what's the alternative?

During my studies in India, I learned a simple breathing technique that lets you control when you push the emergency button. I will cover this method in detail later in the book, but for now I will point out that most of us take very shallow, upper-chest breaths all day long–letting just enough air in and out to get through the day. These shallow breaths stimulate the stress receptors that predominate in the upper lobes of the lungs, triggering the survival stress response. By contrast, the nerves in the lower lobes of the lungs are predominantly supplied with calming and rejuvenating receptors. When you consider that we take between 24,000 and 28,000 breaths every day, you will understand that the kinds of breaths you take, and the areas of the lungs that are stimulated, can have an enormous impact on how you feel and function. By following my simple directions later, you will learn how to take 28,000 calming and restorative, fat-burning breaths during all aspects of your daily life.

Applying these principles of breathing to exercise, I will show you how to make certain that you burn fat as fuel during exercise by never triggering the survival response. I have proven that during vigorous levels of activity, you can reproduce the same kind of alpha and coherent brainwave state reached through meditation or the Relaxation Response. Imagine running as fast as your legs can carry you while your nervous system responds as if it were in meditation! I call this experience the Hurricane Effect.

STRESS AND THE EYE OF THE HURRICANE

When we observe nature, which has been successfully sustaining life for billions of years, we can readily perceive a formula in many of its activities. Earlier I mentioned the hurricane, one of nature's more formidable forces. Viewed from above, a hurricane looks like a giant doughnut, with swirling, gale force winds and clouds wrapped around a fairly calm, cloudless center known as the "eye," which may stretch as much as 60 miles in diameter. The bigger the eye of the hurricane, the more powerful its winds. Although a hurricane's winds can be destructive, they also perform invaluable work transporting water from the Caribbean to the mainland to water our crops and help prevent drought. In much the same fashion, the calmer your nervous system remains through the day, the more productive you can be. Athletes talk about "runner's high," saying that their best race was their easiest race. When two opposite forces coexist in nature, the potential energy is unlimited. From the tiniest atom, in which spinning electrons orbit a silent nucleus, to the sun at the center of nine orbiting planets, to galaxies consisting of billions of suns spiraling around a central core, this formula of stillness and energy in dynamic coexistence demonstrates the universal rhythms of the cosmos.

Nature has cycles that regulate seasons, harvests, migrations, and mating patterns. Every detail is organized in a way that simultaneously supports both the individual and the whole. Survival in nature depends on living in harmony with those cycles—not only for birds and animals but for us as well. Unfortunately, we have insulated ourselves from these cycles and have chosen a way of life that goes dangerously against the natural grain. Plenty of things can happen in our lives that are stressful, but when nature is on our side and our life is flowing in sync with its cycles, rather than working against them, stress does not have the same impact.

Sadly, we have all but lost the sense of calm at the center of vast energy represented by the hurricane. The silence and peace that we all have experienced in a forest or on a mountaintop has been squeezed out of our lives by continuous stress. Without that experience of calm at our hub, we have pushed ourselves beyond our limits and as a result, stress-related chronic diseases have gained a beachhead in the war against our health. As I indicated earlier, recent studies have shown that stress is the cause of at least 80 percent of all disease. Eighty percent! Over the last 20 years, I have seen more than 30,000 patients, and increasingly the most common conditions I am asked to treat are depression and fatigue—the classic symptoms of excessive stress. This is a serious problem in America that will not be solved with antidepressants and stimulants, whether herbal or pharmaceutical. Commercial stress-reduction techniques all attempt to deal with stress after it has already occurred and the damage has been done. My approach seeks to prevent stress before it arises.

Studies also indicate that the most detrimental stressors to our body are not catastrophic events like having your house burn down or losing a loved one. Rather they are the smaller stressful things we do every day of our lives, whose cumulative destructive force is greater than any single traumatic event. If your life runs against the grain of nature for 30 years, it is nearly impossible not to show the wear and tear. As we grow older we watch our eyes go bad in our forties and our joints stiffen up in our fifties, yet we chalk it all up to the aging process. It is nothing of the sort. I believe that physical degeneration is very much the result of living with no connection to the cycles of nature. Many of us are paddling upstream, with huge amounts of stress hitting us head-on. When you're always paddling upstream, you don't need to be hit by a log to be stopped; your arms will eventually get exhausted and you simply won't be able to paddle anymore.

The one unassailable fact that modern science has unearthed about weight loss and gain is that stress is also the major cause of weight gain. On a simple psychological level, stress can lead us to overeat as a way of assuaging our feelings of nervousness, apprehension, fatigue, and low self-worth. We may feel that because we are under such intense time pressure, we just don't have enough time to prepare nutritious meals and eat them in a leisurely, healthful way. On a more complex physiological level, stress involuntarily sets into motion a chain of events that causes the body to gain weight and undergo certain other processes that are deleterious to our health, as I will explain in detail later.

But stress is an integral part of modern life, you may reply. Getting and holding a job that pays well enough to support you, raising a family in an increasingly violent and fragmented world, owning a home, living in a big city, or living in the suburbs and commuting to work—all are inevitable sources of stress. That's certainly true, and although you can seek out ways to minimize that kind of stress in your life, you probably won't be able to remove it altogether, short of joining a religious order and moving to a monastery or ashram. What you can do, however, is reduce the overall level of stress on your system by eating and exercising in the stress-free ways I outline in this book.

DIET AND EXERCISE DAILY STRESS TEST

You can identify the signs of stress derived from eating and exercising in ways that trigger the "survival response" by taking my simple Daily Stress

Test. To determine whether there's room for you to reduce the amount of stress related to diet and exercise, answer the following questions by circling either Yes, No, or Sometimes. (If this is a library book, please copy these next few pages, or use a pencil, lightly, and erase when you've finished.)

1. Are you stiffer in the morning than when you went to bed the night before? Yes No Sometimes
2. Do you drink coffee in the morning to get started? Yes No Sometimes
3. Do you work through lunch so you can leave early? Yes No Sometimes
4. Do you crave coffee, cola, candy, sweets, or a nap in the afternoon? Yes No Sometimes
5. Do you leave work feeling exhausted? Yes No Sometimes
6. Do you normally sit down and have a nice, large dinner in the evening? Yes No Sometimes
7. Do you regularly eat dinner after 8:00 P.M.? Yes No Sometimes
8. Do you eat watching TV, opening mail, reading, or driving? Yes No Sometimes
9. Do you crave breads, pasta, and starches? Yes No Sometimes
10. Do you often suffer from indigestion? Yes No Sometimes
11. Do you get a second wind at 10:00 P.M. and stay up past midnight? Yes No Sometimes
12. Do you often have restless sleep or insomnia? Yes No Sometimes
13. Do you often have difficulty getting up in the morning and tend to feel sleepy all day? Yes No Sometimes
14. Have you tried exercising to lose weight within the past 3 years and given up? Yes No Sometimes
15. Have you tried exercising to lose weight and gained weight instead? Yes No Sometimes
16. Are you too busy to exercise on a regular basis? Yes No Sometimes
17. Do you exercise at lunchtime? Yes No Sometimes
18. Do you hate to exercise? Yes No Sometimes
19. Do you tend toward worry, anxiety, or depression? Yes No Sometimes

20. Have you noticed a marked decline in your sex drive?
    Yes No Sometimes
21. Do you have chronic physical complaints not related to overuse or injuries? Yes No Sometimes
22. Do you often have difficulty remembering things?
    Yes No Sometimes
23. Have you recently noticed your vision deteriorating?
    Yes No Sometimes

Score 2 points for each Yes, 1 point for Sometimes, and 0 for No. If you scored between 0 and 5, your life is in remarkable balance. If your score is between 5 and 15, you are experiencing moderate levels of stress. If your score is between 15 and 20, you may be experiencing stress-related symptoms. If your score is over 20, chances are that stress is a dominant force in your daily existence. In that case, this book will show you how to recapture the eye of the hurricane–the sense of peace and calm in the midst of activity.

In the course of this book, I will address each of the questions above and show you how you can eat, exercise, and enjoy your life while making it *less* stressful, not more. Following these suggestions most of the time will yield huge dividends in your health and well-being. Once you experience life in harmony with nature, you will never go back to any other way of living. As I recommend the changes to your daily regimen of eating and exercise, try them, but remember my golden rule: If you don't like it, don't do it, because if you don't like something you will not stick with it.

IT'S NOT JUST WHAT YOU EAT, BUT WHEN AND HOW

About 13 years ago, I went for my first consultation with an Ayurvedic physician. When I arrived, his nurse took my blood pressure, and to my surprise it was high: 135 over 95 (the normal range is 110–120 over 70–80). I was so surprised that I had the nurse try three different blood pressure cuffs, on both arms, but the results always came back the same. I was only 27 years old, I exercised every day, ate good food, meditated, and thought I lived a relatively stress-free life. I could only imagine that

I must have some congenital ailment that I'd been unaware of. Then the doctor walked in, looked at me, grabbed my wrist, and took my pulse. Ayurvedic physicians are trained to take the pulse in a much different fashion from Western doctors, and as a result they garner much more detailed information from it. The doctor began by asking me what I ate for lunch. I told him I ate a big breakfast and a big dinner, but didn't usually have much for lunch. I had a busy practice and lunch was always small, quick, and eaten on the run. He told me to go home and have a large, hot, relaxing lunch in the middle of the day, adding that if I did this every day, I would never have high blood pressure again.

I thought the man was crazy. How in the world could lunch have anything to do with my high blood pressure? But out of sheer curiosity I eventually started to follow his advice. Since then I have never taken any medication for my blood pressure, and yet thirteen years later, with five kids, a busy practice, a radio program, and dozens of speaking engagements every year, my blood pressure is stable at 110 over 70. I attribute this principally to one thing: I take one and a half hours for lunch almost every day, and I make it the largest meal of the day. My lunch has become by far the most important part of my personal day, and I do my best not to shortchange myself with a quick bite eaten on the run or while making phone calls.

Before I started following this plan, I used to leave work feeling as if I'd been hit by a truck, a bus, or at least a car. I was exhausted and stressed out. If I did not exercise or meditate as soon as I got home, I would carry that stress into the evening, which felt terrible. I am convinced that this is the reason people drink alcohol after work and crave big dinners. If the body is not satisfied at lunch, it will strain through the afternoon and crave an emotional meal or drink at night. When I changed my eating habits, not only did my blood pressure level off, but that feeling of being exhausted and stressed after work disappeared as well—and I lost weight! I can honestly say that I now typically leave work with the same energy and clarity of mind as when I started my day.

In fact, this has become the easiest way for me to monitor how I am handling stress: If I leave work strained and tense, the first thing I look at is how and when I am eating, and then I go about fixing that. It is normal not to be exhausted at the end of a hard day's work, unless, of course, you were digging ditches all day. I have given the same recommendation to literally thousands of people over the years and have seen miracles, and not just with their blood pressure. As I will show in more detail in chapter 6, the remaining piece of the 3-Season Diet program concerns not *what* you eat, but when and how you eat it. Even if you have a full day balancing family and career, I'll have plenty of practical suggestions for making the big lunch a part of your life.

A FINAL WORD ABOUT CRAVINGS

To achieve a balanced diet without overeating, we have to learn how to develop a hunger level that is governed by appropriate desires and cravings. Through my research and practice with thousands of patients, I have determined that if your body craves something, it actually needs what it craves—even if that something is inappropriate and ultimately unhealthful! The problem is not the craving but the imbalance that has led to the craving, as we will see in the next chapter when we examine the fad diets of the past century. As you learn to shift your diet into alignment with the seasons, your body will learn to crave foods that are appropriate for each time of year. Once you have returned to a natural balance of eating, your hunger level will determine how much you should or shouldn't eat, and simple shopping lists that you can hang on the refrigerator door will guide you to the best foods to buy for each season. Later in the book I will include a listing of all the foods harvested around the world that are appropriate to eat in winter, summer, or spring. For example, although only nuts and grains and some root vegetables and starches are available in winter in the northern United States, you will be able to enjoy bananas and avocados and other heavier, winter-balancing fruits and greens harvested in the winter in other parts of the world.

People who attended weeklong rejuvenation workshops at my LifeSpa in Colorado have reported wonderful changes in their appetite. They still have passionate cravings for certain foods, but the foods they crave have changed. In winter, when the body is building its natural fat supplies, they now crave soups and nuts, warm grains, and other protein-rich foods, as well as meat and fish if they desire. They crave salads and leafy greens in spring, as their appetite naturally diminishes and they cleanse themselves from their heavy winter repast with a naturally occurring low-fat diet. And they crave fruit, starches, pastas, and other high-energy, high-carb foods in summer, when they are most physically active. They have learned to live according to nature's design.

Combining the 3-Season Diet with my revolutionary approach to exercise will help you achieve and maintain your ideal weight without feeling like a martyr to the cause. Stress and misguided eating habits have stripped the natural calm and silence from our bodies at the cellular level. This book will help you return calm and serenity to your daily life and gain access to your full human potential. If you follow my simple instructions about eating the foods most appropriate for each season, adjusting the diet according to your body type, eating the majority of your food at the optimum time of day, and exercising in such a way that your body does not perceive it as a survival situation, you will not only lose excess pounds and maintain your ideal weight. You will also live in the calm eye of the hurricane, remaining serene even as you generate undreamed of energy and power in your daily life. And you will never need another diet book again.

CHAPTER 2

The Diet-Go-Round

FOR MUCH OF THIS century we have struggled from one diet to the next, none of them lasting more than a few years and none succeeding in their one universally trumpeted goal: to help people lose weight and keep it off. There's a good reason for this dilemma: *Each diet that has come along has merely been a response to the nutritional imbalance created by previous fad diets, without addressing the underlying problems!* I realized how the "newest best-selling diet" provided only symptomatic relief for the previous diet's shortcomings after talking to my Aunt Jo-Anne.

AUNT JO-ANNE'S INSIGHT

As I was preparing to write this book, I called my Aunt Jo-Anne, who had always had trouble controlling her weight. Like so many Americans, she has tried each of the popular diets in succession as it came along. Twenty-seven years ago, after giving birth to two sons, my aunt was unable to lose the weight she had gained during her pregnancies and had gone on a high-protein diet, which she laughingly referred to as "the cottage cheese and hamburger diet." All she could remember about it was her constant craving for breads, pasta, potatoes, and doughnuts. That started her on a succession of diets, none of which helped her to keep off the weight she lost from them. Now in her late forties, however, she has finally discerned the pattern that defeats her. "It seems that every time I go on a diet," she told me, "I end up craving more and more of the food I'm not supposed to eat on that ridiculous diet!"

If she was on a low-fat diet, for instance, after a time of faithfully following its rules Aunt Jo-Anne would crave nuts, oil, red meat, and cheese. If it was a sugar-free diet, she would stick to it for a few months but end up dreaming about chocolates, ice cream, cookies, and cake. After she had shed the 20 or 30 pounds she had set out to lose, she would go off the diet and almost unconsciously start to binge on the very foods she had been deprived of. Voilà! The weight would return, and then some. Aunt Jo-Anne would become so frustrated that she would try eating less, but she only succeeded in starving herself and adding to her growing anxiety around food. As her frustration and anxiety mounted, she would begin looking for another diet. "This time," Jo-Anne lamented, "I would look for one that would allow me to eat what I'd been craving, and still lose weight."

Some doctor, nutritionist, or researcher would be only too happy to provide the next diet that would appear to solve the dilemma faced by Jo-Anne—and just about every other person in America who had been following the previous diet. So after Jo-Anne had given up fatty foods for a year or more, along came a diet telling her that she could eat those foods as long as she first ate a grapefruit, for example, or as long as she ate only large amounts of protein and stayed away from carbohydrates.

As my aunt spoke, I realized why people who are dieting all the time can't seem to lose weight, or to keep it off once they lose it. Suddenly I understood how as a nation we had gone from the "miracle" of a high-protein diet 27 years ago to the latest weight-loss "miracle"—the high-protein diet—and still had an obesity rate that is the highest in the world. Nobody seems to ask why, if such a diet didn't work back then, and was followed by a rapid succession of equally restrictive diets that also failed, this same diet should work today. And yet it probably will work—for a year or two, until the craving for the foods that it restricts overcomes the most heroic willpower in the world and dieters start bingeing once again on what they need.

When Charlene came to see me, she had grown from a size 6 to a size 22. While aggressively trying to lose weight over the past 2 years, she had actually *gained* 105 pounds. She had first begun dieting after a gain of 20 pounds left her weighing 135. An emergency room nurse in Boulder, Colorado, Charlene sought out a diet according to the medical model based on the latest research. Nonetheless, she soon found herself going from one diet to another. Each diet would typically allow her to shed some of the original weight gain, but not long after losing the weight she would invariably gain it all back—with an additional 5 or 10 pounds. After 2 years of this she weighed 220 and was frustrated and depressed.

Charlene was consistently told to eat a low-fat diet, avoiding fatty meats, nuts, and oils. When her willpower finally failed her, she would consume not just nuts and oils but pastries, chips, and other high-fat foods that caused her weight to balloon. I put Charlene on a seasonal diet rich in natural fats (for example, more fish and chicken, nuts, oils, and grains) and gave her pointers on how and when to eat. In a very short time her excess weight began to fall off, and she said that she never felt hungry or deprived.

I can't emphasize enough that if you feel like you are starving, you probably are. During starvation, the body does its best to store fat and burn emergency fuel, primarily sugar and simple carbs. Each time we fall into the cycle of starvation dieting, craving, bingeing, and dieting again, we are training our bodies to store fat (meaning to add weight) and burn the fuel that it normally saves for emergencies. We have been killing ourselves for the better part of the last century trying to lose weight without any long-term success. The body cannot successfully be *forced* to lose weight, because it will always respond to restrictive diets in a rebound fashion, craving whatever the diet lacked.

Some popular weight-loss programs—like the new high-protein diets—are designed to force the body into fat metabolism by depriving it of carbohydrates. With no ready source of energy from carbs, the body will be *forced* to burn fat for fuel. You do begin to lose weight, but it is as a result of carbohydrate starvation. Studies at MIT have shown that the inevitable result of restricting the diet in this extreme fashion is eventual bingeing on carbs to such an extent that the body gains back all the weight it has lost and more. That's why I have designed my 3-Season eating plan (along with my weight-balancing program) so that you will not find yourself craving one particular food group, whether it's fats, carbs, sugars, or proteins, because that would only result in storing fat and craving more food.

Looking back over the most popular diets that have appeared since the end of the Second World War, I discovered that each one lasted from two to five years at most before it was replaced by something new. Many years later, with a face-lift and some modernization, these once-disproven diets would again surge to the top of the charts and be touted as the newest and greatest diet around. If this sounds incredible to you, it may help to take a brief look at some of these diets and how they worked—or failed to work. In the process, we'll gain a more complete knowledge of how our bodies respond to food.

LOW-CALORIE, THE FIRST LOW-FAT DIET

Calories are units of heat based on the energy-producing quality of food; proteins, carbohydrates, and sugars all have varying levels of calories. If the heat energy derived from food is not burned off, or if the amount of calories consumed is simply too much for the body to metabolize between mealtimes, the excess calories will be stored as fat. In an agricultural society where people spent long days toiling in the fields, they burned off most of the calories from the food they ate, especially when it was consumed early in the day. The lower physical demands of our largely sedentary life have conspired with the abundance and constant availability of food—especially food that is increasingly processed and indigestible—to produce the epidemic of overweight and obesity in this country. The first and seemingly most logical approach to losing weight, therefore, is simply to consume fewer calories.

To help dieters to this end, low-calorie foods proliferated in the 1950s and '60s; as America became obsessed with counting calories, caloric measurements began to be required for food and beverage labels. When you reduce calories, however, you also reduce the fuel necessary to produce sufficient energy for the tasks of the day. The body responds to this depletion of energy stores as a survival situation, and, as we have seen, resorts to storing fat for the long haul and burning emergency fuel in the form of sugar. When the body says, "I need fuel now," we crave sugar or a stimulant in some form because it is metabolized so quickly in the mouth and stomach and we don't have to wait until it gets very far in the 30-foot-long processing plant known as the human digestive tract. But precisely because the form of energy created by burning sugar is intense and short lived, the net result is that dieters experience brief rushes of energy followed by a feeling of letdown or burnout. Somewhat like drug addicts living for that next "hit" of speed or cocaine, dieters need more of a "fix" each time. They then begin to crave the very foods they have been lacking, namely fats, to replenish the feeling of comfort and satiety that only fat can provide.

This explains why the first dieters so often went off their low-calorie diets and wound up overeating to make up for the starvation of the diet program, as my Aunt Jo-Anne had so astutely observed. After they gained back the weight they had lost and more, they would often try to police their own eating habits, imposing ad hoc starvation diets in a valiant attempt to get their weight back down to where it had been at the peak of their dietary success. But because their bodies had been conditioned to burn sugar for energy and store fat, they would paradoxically put on more weight. As their failure to keep off the weight increased their stress levels, dieters would eventually decide that they needed to go on another formal diet.

Food itself became the enemy, and dieters entered into a love-hate relationship with the nation's abundant food supply. Far from being perceived as a pleasurable and relaxing reward for hard work, eating became associated with guilt and stress. Like alcoholics or drug addicts who often feel guilty even as they rush to satisfy their hunger for more stimulation, overeaters entered into a vicious spiral of starvation, bingeing, guilt, and shame. Since relying on willpower to eat less was torture for most people, when a new diet came along offering a solution to the previous diet's failure, dieters would jump on the bandwagon out of desperation. And so the infamous yo-yo diet syndrome was born.

THE LOW-FAT DIET

The low-calorie diet was actually a forerunner of the classic low-fat diet, since it stressed lowering the consumption of highly caloric fats by eating chicken without the skin, or the leanest cuts of meet, or cottage cheese instead of higher-fat cheddar or brie. By eliminating excess fats, along with sugar and even certain simple carbohydrates such as chips and bread, dieters could lower their caloric intake significantly. This approach has been followed with certain variations by Weight Watchers, Jenny Craig, and other formal diet systems that all rely on the basic principles first espoused in the low-calorie, low-fat diets of the 1950s and '60s. Eliminating fat was quite a task, however, because fat was everywhere in the American diet. During the early postwar years, steak, hamburgers, french fries, shakes, malteds, ice cream, milk, and butter were nutritional mainstays.

FAKE FAT

To combat the pervasive menace of fat and sugar, science and the food industry worked together to create a series of artificial products that mimicked the taste qualities of the real things while eliminating their caloric impact. One of the first fruits of their research was the development of a synthetic process that could convert liquid vegetable oils to solid fats by adding hydrogen. The result was oleomargarine, which functioned like butter but had absolutely no animal fat—the so-called bad fat. At first margarine was unpopular because of its poor taste and visual appeal, largely because the dairy industry, wary of competition, insisted that margarine be white to distinguish it from butter. But during the 1940s and '50s, margarine manufacturers supported a number of state initiatives, or popular ballots, to allow their product to be yellow. With the addition of artificial flavor, and a dizzying array of television and print ads to promote this new "miracle" food, margarine became enormously popular. Any self-respecting, health-conscious American knew that fat was bad for you and so would choose synthetic margarine over real butter, based on its presumed ability to reduce fat in the diet.

It was several decades before studies came out that disproved the miraculous claims of the margarine manufacturers. We now know that the process of hydrolysis creates margarine by turning polyunsaturated fats into saturated or "trans fats," which do not occur in nature and are actually hazardous to health. According to the *Journal of Nutrition*, the trans fats in margarine have been shown to *raise* cholesterol levels in humans. The British *Journal of Preventative Social Medicine* reported that people who eat high amounts of margarine or any hydrogenated oils have a greater risk of heart disease.

Hydrogenated vegetable oils, produced by a similar process but retaining their liquid state, were marketed as the next scientific "miracle." These processed oils would not turn rancid, as natural oils do when exposed to air over time, and could therefore sit on the shelf in a jar of peanut butter or mayonnaise and virtually never separate or go bad, even without refrigeration. New brands of peanut butter made with partially hydrogenated oils, like Skippy and Jif (even the names implied speed and convenience) not only lasted longer on the shelf but also came in homogenized form, without the inconvenience of having to stir up the oil that separated out of traditional peanut butter. Manufacturers even added sugar to their products to make them more appetizing to kids, ignoring the extra calories that came with it. (Today, McDonald's adds sugar to their fries for the same reason. Any teenager will tell you that McDonald's makes the best fries—their sugar-salt combo is the secret.) Potato chips would be limp if it were not for the hydrogenated oils in them, which also account for their high levels of fat and cholesterol. Unfortunately, partially hydrogenated oils make food less digestible, and the oxidation of the fat in these undigestible oils is a major cause of high cholesterol levels in the body.

DIET SUGAR

At the same time that margarine and hydrogenated oils were being invented, scientists were actively researching ways to produce an artificial sweetener that could replace sugar. Saccharin had been around since 1879, but now there was a real call for its use, and it became the first of several inexpensive substances introduced to the marketplace that did not have the chemical properties of sugar but that did taste sweet—about 350 times as sweet as sucrose. Soon saccharin was being used as a sugar replacement to sweeten just about every high-cal item on the American menu, allowing dieters to consume all the bad stuff they had been told to avoid, from cola drinks, coffee, and tea to chewing gum, cake, and Popsicles, without fear of gaining weight.

These sugar-free products now had no calories, but they also produced no real energy, because the energy had come from the sugar. The illusion of energy that dieters associated with the sweet taste, however, provided at least a short-lived feeling of satisfaction. Besides, cola, coffee, and tea were all laced with caffeine, which provided a real, if fleeting, burst of energy similar to that of sugar. Saccharin did help people lose weight in the beginning, although the sugar-free era also spawned some problems that are still to be unraveled more than 30 years later. Saccharin, for instance, has been shown to act as a carcinogen in rats, although it continues to be marketed as an alternative sweetener. Artificial sweeteners called cyclamates came and went fairly quickly, being banned in the United States in 1969 because of health safety issues; nonetheless, an attempt is under way to reintroduce cyclamates here.

The more recent alternative sweetener, aspartame, marketed as NutraSweet, has been extensively studied, and although test results have been largely favorable, there have been enough anecdotal accounts of negative responses to aspartame to raise doubts. Aspartame is an amino acid that is a stimulant to the body, and some users have linked it to overstimulation in children, leading to attention deficit disorder (ADD), as well as to migraine headaches and depression. Bad as those sugary soft drinks are for you, the dietetic alternatives could be even worse. In my clinical practice, I have seen remarkable improvements in kids diagnosed with ADD (attention deficit disorder) or ADHD (attention deficit with hyperactivity disorder) by taking them off all NutraSweet products. We know that refined white sugar is toxic to the human body; among other things, it leaches B vitamins from the nervous system. Yet because sugar has not been proven to be a carcinogen, even white refined sugar in small amounts in certain instances is still preferable to saccharin. Unfortunately, many people have become hypersensitive to sugar and are now forced to use artificial sweeteners. I will address this issue more in chapter 9. (Alternative products that resemble the natural footprint of sugar cane have recently begun appearing on the market. Societies that eat natural sugar cane have pearly white teeth and perfectly normal sugar and fat metabolism. Raw sugar, cane sugar, honey, and other natural sweeteners remain your best bet, especially when used in moderation.)

Not surprisingly, the afternoon energy surge built on sugar-free drinks, caffeine, high-carb snacks, and in many cases nicotine as well, not only wore off by five o'clock but left you feeling more depleted than before.

Like a small-scale version of a cocaine high or adrenaline rush, the caffeine that remained in coffee and cola drinks after the sugar was removed got you wired but provided no follow-up energy. When the buzz wore off, you tended to feel strung out—and you were! Soon the body began to crave "real" food, and once again dieters fell off the wagon, bingeing on fats, sugars, and carbs to make up for the lack of natural energy.

But now something even more insidious was beginning to happen to the diet-crazed and still-overweight public. As the "fake sugar" regimen increasingly supplanted any sense of satisfying, nutritionally balanced meals eaten at leisure, the natural blood sugar regulation of the body became extremely fragile. The term "hypoglycemia" was coined to describe this dire new syndrome of chronic low blood sugar levels. Being hypoglycemic is a little like driving an automobile with half a gallon of gas in the tank and a tendency to stall, but having only enough money to buy one gallon of gas at a time. The result is that you have to keep pulling over to refuel and are never sure how long you can go between stops. This problem has yet to be totally remedied by any new diet.

THE DIET ONSLAUGHT

The binge-rebound cravings that dieters experienced were typically so strong that their low-sugar and low-fat foods went out the window and they began to consume food with an excess of fat and sugar. Suffering through a low-fat diet for 6 months or more, losing 10 to 30 pounds only to gain it all back after falling off the diet, was a depressing experience. After many dieters landed back where they had started, they were even more determined than ever to lose weight but were wary of any diet requiring them to starve themselves. A number of gimmicky diets now began to appear in fairly rapid succession, offering "miraculous" results similar to the low-cal, low-fat diets but without the martyrdom. The Hollywood Grapefruit Diet, for instance, promised that you could eat anything you wanted, including fat and sugar, as long as you ate a grapefruit before each meal. It banked on the antioxidant properties of the grapefruit to break down the "bad" fats that cause high cholesterol levels and weight gain, while still providing the satiety of a traditional American meal high in fat and sugar. Grapefruits have been shown over the years to be loaded with vitamin C, a powerful antioxidant, and more recently grapefruit seed extracts have been proven to have both antimicrobial and antioxidant qualities. Antioxidants such as vitamins C and E are believed to scavenge the system for free radicals, a prime cause of aging, disease, and weight gain. Unfortunately, even the mysterious power of the grapefruit antioxidants was not strong enough to mitigate the fat-storing effects of stress, processed and refined foods, and overeating.

HIGH-PROTEIN DIETS

Around this time, in the early 1970s, Dr. Robert C. Atkins came out with a striking alternative to the low-cal, low-fat regimen: the high-protein diet. This diet had actually been in use as far back as the 1860s, when an English casket maker named William Banting introduced it. Other variations on the diet included Dr. Herman Taller's *Calories Don't Count* in 1961, and *The Doctor's Quick Weight-Loss Diet* by Dr. Irwin Stillman. All these diets are based on the fact that one way to lower the amount of fat and sugar you eat is to increase your intake of lean protein. Because, as we will see, the fats in high-protein foods tend to leave one feeling full, dieters don't get as hungry between meals. Since many people's favorite foods—meat, poultry, fish, and dairy products—contain protein, this diet was and continues to be enormously appealing.

Not only is protein absolutely essential for health, but excess protein in the diet is rarely stored as fat, being processed out of the body through the urine as uric acid, and so does not contribute to weight gain. (In extreme amounts, protein can cause gout, long known as the "rich man's disease" because protein is the most expensive form of food, but this is relatively rare today.) A high-protein diet—which is really a low-carb (low-energy) diet—promotes weight loss because it forces the body into fat metabolism. You have to get your energy somewhere, and in this case the fat stores are the only place the body has to go. Weight lifters have long known that if they wanted to strip away the fat from around the muscles and prepare for bodybuilding competitions, in which each individual muscle in the body seems to want to reach out and touch someone, they should eat nothing but protein for two weeks prior to competition.

But protein does not provide much energy, and this diet restricts carbohydrates that do, so it leaves dieters feeling dull and listless. As with all restrictive diets, people eventually longed for those energy-producing foods like bread, pasta, fruit juice, and sweets that were forbidden them. Even mainstream publications have begun to catch on to the counter-productive aspects of the high-protein diet. Writing in the *New York Times* in 1999, Jane Brody explained, "Because carbohydrates hold water in the body, as your body becomes depleted of stored carbohydrates, the first five pounds or so you lose on this plan is not fat weight but water, quickly regained with the first starchy food eaten." Once again, dieters ran the risk of gaining more weight than they had lost in the first place. A number of nutritional researchers have also had harsh words for high-protein diets in general. Miriam Nelson of Tufts University warns that the diets "may cause dizziness and extreme fatigue." Dr. Charles Baum of the University of Illinois cautions against the loss of essential miner-als from the bones and elevated lipid levels caused by the increased intake of animal fat. But the main problem is that because it restricts so many foods that people instinctively enjoy, including fruits, vegetables, and pasta, the diet generates a feeling of dissatisfaction that causes dieters to give it up.

HIGH-CARB DIETS

In the 1970s and '80s, as people were seeking a remedy for the low energy created by low-carb, high-protein diets, the dietary pendulum took a pro-nounced swing away from protein and toward expanding consumption of complex carbohydrates. High-protein diets were not working and people were already bingeing on carbs, so, predictably, a new diet emerged that gave people permission to eats plenty of carbs and get their energy back, while losing weight into the bargain. High-carb diets were also a response to the rapidly growing blood sugar problems created by stress and the vacillation between sugar-free substitutes and cravings for sugar as well as a growing inability to metabolize fat for energy. Popular books like *Eat to Win* and *The Pritikin Diet* proposed reducing fat intake while recommending that as much as 70 to 80 percent of the diet be composed of complex carbs. Much of the theoretical backing for high carbs came from studies of Third World countries, where the population could not afford to eat protein. They ate diets high in carbohydrates such as rice, millet, quinoa, corn, fruits, and vegetables, and reported much lower levels of heart disease and cancer than their richer, protein-consuming counterparts.

What the studies failed to take into account was that the populations of these countries lived radically different lives that more closely resembled the agricultural standard of our ancestors than the industrial model of our own time. The grains they ate were also generally whole and unrefined, still containing all their vital proteins and fats. And although we in the Northern Hemisphere tend to associate Third World life with the constant stress of poverty, the day-to-day lives of many of those people were far less stressful and more involved with family support systems than our own hectic and highly alienated lives.

The high-carb, low-fat diet is healthy, to be sure, promoting high fiber and roughage intake while deriving energy from complex carbohydrates like pasta and vegetables, which tend to burn more slowly than the simple carbohydrates in bread, chips, and crackers. But with stress levels in our culture rising and the body being fed only complex carbs and low-fat foods, the body soon becomes deficient in the so-called good fats: essential fatty acids that provide the fuel for hormones, cellular metabolism, and a host of other necessary functions. In a high-stress world, eating a diet composed of 70 percent complex carbs will send a message to the sugar-burning engines to rev up and forget about burning fat for energy. Complex carbs may be slow burning, but they are still sugars, as all carbohydrates are in essence. If you do not give the body fat to burn for at least 4 months of the year—during winter, when the body especially needs the fat for insulation and to generate more heat—the body will gradually replace its ability to metabolize fat as fuel with a tendency to burn sugars.

It is more than a coincidence that after 5 years of high-carb diets, cholesterol levels were suddenly going off the charts. Studies have shown conclusively that when the body is metabolizing extremely high amounts of sugar for long periods of time, insulin levels are unnaturally high. This not only tells the body not to burn fat, but also directs it to make more cholesterol as a response to the need to create more stress-fighting hormones made from cholesterol. As a result, on the heels of high-carb diets during the 1970s and '80s, the focus of attention shifted from fat to cholesterol, the fatlike substance in the bloodstream produced by the liver but also absorbed from some foods. Although cholesterol is essential to the production of cell membranes and certain hormones, the body already makes all the cholesterol it needs. When excess amounts are absorbed from fatty foods, they accumulate on arterial walls, producing plaque, which stiffens arteries and reduces their ability to handle changes in blood pressure. Plaque also narrows the space through which blood can pass in the arteries, forcing the heart to work harder. When enough plaque accumulates, it can totally block blood flow or rupture and create clots, leading to heart attack or stroke.

LOW-CHOLESTEROL DIETS

As the public became increasingly aware of this chemistry, cholesterol-lowering diets to save our cardiovascular systems became popular. These were actually sophisticated low-fat diets that did seem to work for a while, especially for people who already suffered from heart disease. Perhaps the most popular of the low-fat, low-cholesterol diets was proposed by Dr. Dean Ornish, whose cleansing and healing regimen combined very low levels of fat and lots of carbs. Although Dr. Ornish does allow his clients to eat small amounts of very lean meat, his is essentially a vegetarian diet. Along with this low-fat regimen, Ornish prescribed yoga and meditation to help reduce the stress in our culture that is the primary cause of weight gain, an admirable goal.

The low-fat tactic works fine for anybody suffering from heart disease, along with those at risk due to hereditary or physiological predisposition. But a diet that cleans you out and restores balance is not necessarily something you should continue year in and year out. Once fat returns to normal levels, there is a danger that this diet can render the body deficient in fat. It is no accident that a deficiency of essential fatty acids is believed by some experts to be one of the most common causes of allergies and depression. Removing fats from the diet to such an extent can also make it difficult for any but the most highly motivated dieters—heart attack victims, for instance— to stick with such a plan. Raw green salads are certainly healthy, but substituting lemon juice for the oils that give salads their appetizing appeal makes it difficult for most people to stick with the program.

Eating low-fat or fat-free foods can also give dieters an illusory sense that they won't gain weight, when what really matters is not fat content but calories. "People assumed that if a food had no fat, they could eat as much of it as they wanted," Dr. Alice H. Lichtenstein, a professor of nutrition at Tufts University in Boston, told the *New York Times*. "But many low-fat and fat-free products have nearly as many calories as their full-fat versions. Reducing fat alone is no guarantee of weight loss. You must cut calories or increase physical activity."

THE ALTERNATIVE DIETS

I don't want to give the impression that the commercial high-protein, high-carb, and low-fat diets were the only ones on the market during the last half century. A number of natural weight-control systems, ranging from the traditional Japanese diet known as macrobiotics to the ancient practice of vegetarianism, which reaches back at least to the first millennium B.C. in India, enjoyed relatively low popularity but did offer useful alternatives to the mainstream diets.

Proponents of the Macrobiotic Diet insist that all food be cooked, because cooking tends to make food more digestible by helping to break it down in advance. Advocates of a Raw Food Diet, such as Norman Walker and Ann Wigmore, represent the opposing view that to gain the most nutritional value from food, we ought to eat it in its raw or "live" state, without any cooking. At the Hippocrates Institute in Palm Beach, Florida, you won't find a stove or even a toaster. Wigmore and her followers not only eat fruits and vegetables in their raw state, they also grow their own sprouted beans, seeds, and fresh wheat grass, which they press into a dark, pungent liquid that tastes a little like molten garlic but is a potent food for cleansing and good health.

The Wigmore regimen draws on the concept that seeds and nuts provide the unadulterated core of life, which nutritionist Bernie Jensen has long promoted in this country but which is universally accepted in the East. When I was studying in India, the Ayurvedic masters spoke of "the sweet heart of the coconut." When a coconut ripens and falls from the tree, the moment it hits the sand it begins to germinate a seed within it, potentially to create a new coconut tree. The water in the center of that green coconut begins to congeal into a core the size of a lacrosse ball and the consistency of a fresh marshmallow. Eventually, that core will liquefy into milk, but the medicinal properties of the "sweet heart" of the coconut, if harvested in the brief time before it becomes liquid, are believed to be 400 times more potent than fresh coconut milk. This enhanced potency occurs with all sprouted grains, seeds, nuts, and legumes and is why sprouts are such an important, naturally occurring food for the spring. The raw-food concept aims to make use of that potency inherent in seeds, nuts, and grasses in their prime as a source of great restorative energy, and advocates eating only the freshest, most recently harvested fruits and vegetables without heating them in any way, which advocates of this diet believe tends to destroy the vital essence of raw foods.

I am strongly in favor of introducing potent raw foods into the diet at the right time, particularly in the spring and summer, and certainly believe in eating the freshest organic produce possible whenever it is available. I would even advise using this diet as a cleansing regime for certain conditions and body types. But as with the Dean Ornish Diet, what cleans out your system and helps correct a particular imbalance is not generally the best diet to help you maintain a balance for the rest of your life. If your car's transmission is slipping, you have to take it to the shop and let the mechanics restore it to good working order, but you don't keep going back to the transmission specialists every week. You may just need to change the oil and rotate the tires every few months to keep your vehicle in good running order.

One dietary tactic that required frequent trips to the market is known as grazing—eating small amounts of food every few hours. Since the body was having trouble processing either large amounts of protein with very little fat, or high carbohydrates with little protein or fat, grazing was proposed as the best way to counteract low-blood sugar. As I toured the country lecturing at fitness industry conventions over the years, I heard many personal trainers and nutritionists recommend grazing for clients who were perfectly healthy. But the problem with grazing is that it acclimates the body to an up-and-down scenario in which it never has quite enough to eat or enough time to digest food completely. It is as if you cooked a pot of rice halfway through, then opened the lid, threw in some more raw rice and cold water, and let it continue to cook. You would end up with a gunky mess of partially cooked rice that nobody could digest. The human digestive system is designed to eat a large meal and fully digest it before taking in substantially more. Depending on your metabolic body type and the fat content of the food consumed, a large meal can take from 1 to 3 hours in the upper digestive tract. By eating in small amounts all day, we never give the digestive system a rest; it is constantly engaged and this is unnatural for the body, which depends on cycles of rest and activity.

The situation is similar to certain rechargeable batteries that laptop computers use: If you recharge the battery before it has run down completely, it soon loses the ability to hold a charge for very long. With enough grazing, the body becomes deconditioned to its accustomed task of digesting a large amount of food and burning it slowly to provide a level stream of energy. It begins to *need* that small feeding every couple of hours, with the result that energy levels remain consistently low. In this way, grazing can sometimes create blood sugar instability in healthy people! And since food is being processed too quickly, the body burns primarily sugars and carbohydrates and stores fat, with the unsurprising result that you gain weight. When the body gets accustomed to small meals every 2 hours and all of a sudden you miss a meal, your blood sugar and energy levels plummet, triggering a resultant craving for more emergency fuel in the form of carbs and sugars—which will create more highs and lows in blood sugar. And those extreme peaks and valleys in blood sugar and insulin levels are again telling the body to save and store fat.

The MacDougal Plan, a favorite of mine, is a vegetarian diet high in starches, fruit, and vegetables, and low in fat—a low-cholesterol regimen that prescribed a ratio of 80 percent carbs, 10 percent protein, and 10 percent fat. Most Americans find it difficult, however, to eat a balanced vegetarian diet. Beans and rice take a long time to prepare properly, and cooking tofu, a major source of protein for vegetarians, requires some practice to create appealing meals. Unfortunately, most who tried the MacDougal Plan failed simply because it didn't fit into our American way of life, given busy schedules and the tempting availability of fast food in restaurants and stores. Even those who stay on a vegetarian diet find it hard not to become protein-deficient and sugar-dependent. It is easy to start eating more sugars and refined carbs that do provide relatively fast-burning energy compared to the steady energy produced by metabolizing fats. Vegetarians often develop strong cravings for sugar and coffee to bolster sagging energy levels.

Variations on the vegetarian theme included the Cabbage Diet, which held that you could eat pretty much whatever you wanted as long as you also consumed lots of cabbage, generally in the form of cabbage soup. Cabbage acts as a diuretic and flushes fat and waste from other foods out of the system, but this does little to raise energy levels or reeducate the body to the wisdom of eating large meals of slow-burning fuel. HerbaLife promised that herbal supplements such as guarana and ephedra *(ma huang)* would stimulate a higher metabolic rate in the body and help burn off fat and calories. This is somewhat akin to taking speed to trick the body into faster metabolism. All during the diet era, some people used coffee and tobacco for the same reason; caffeine and nicotine are both stimulants that tend to depress appetite and stimulate metabolism, although to a lesser extent than amphetamine or benzedrine, the preferred weight-control drugs prior to the 1950s. Have you ever heard someone you know complain that when she finally gave up smoking, she gained 20 pounds? We already know how fatally destructive a nicotine habit can be, but caffeine over time can be almost as debilitating physically, causing headaches, insomnia, and a whole host of digestive difficulties.

COFFEE

Coffee probably deserves a chapter all to itself in any book on nutrition, because it has proven the one constant way that Americans have tried to deal with the low energy levels generated both by the early low-calorie, low-sugar diets and the high-protein, low-carb diets of later years. Madison Avenue fueled demand for coffee by creating massive television ad campaigns for Maxwell House and other popular brands, driving home the message that it was good to drink coffee in the morning for a quick burst of energy. Coffee does stimulate the body and create energy, but it's ultimately a false energy with nothing backing it up. It's a little like borrowing money from the bank to get through the month, but never earning any money to pay back the loan. Eventually, you go into debt and have to file for bankruptcy. Cheap energy not fueled by solid food is the equivalent of cheap credit not backed up by collateral or earning power. (Is it sheer coincidence that the number of personal bankruptcies filed over the past decade has increased exponentially as the populace consistently went into energetic debt?) I find it no surprise that candida, Epstein-Barr virus, chronic fatigue syndrome, and fibromyalgia—all conditions created by stress, which drives the need for the cheap energy of coffee, sugar, and other stimulants—have become so prevalent in recent decades. Our increasing reliance on coffee may also be a factor in the epidemic of clinical depression currently being treated by drugs and herbs ranging from Prozac and Zoloft to Saint-John's-wort.

If coffee had any drawback, it might have been its somewhat lumpen, blue-collar image. The reprise of the low-fat diet in the 1990s, however, helped ring in the runaway success of Starbucks and the next incarnation of coffeemania, this time disguised as chic with dozens of "hip" caffeine drinks, including espresso, cappuccino, *caffè latte*, mocha, and other acceptably exotic coffees. Now along with your caffeine fix you could also pick up a cookie, brownie, or other sugary treat, adding a second instant rush and making these ultra-urban coffee shops little more than legal speed dispensaries.

A traditional place for coffee has nonetheless long existed in the daily routine. In Europe, the time for that cup of espresso or cappuccino is usually after the big midday meal, when the mild amount of caffeine in those drinks stimulates digestion. This helps the body begin to metabolize generous amounts of food and counteracts the tendency to feel drowsy after a big meal. That's a far cry from waking up to two or three cups of coffee in the morning, especially on an empty stomach—and particularly with American coffee that is higher in caffeine, cup for cup, than espresso or cappuccino. Ultimately, coffee is just another classic example of treating symptoms rather than the cause. It has harmonized with the energetic shortcomings of so many of the fad diets of the last century that we could probably call it the perfect counterpoint to insufficient nutrition.

By relying increasingly on cheap, fast energy sources, whether sugars and carbs or caffeine and nicotine, you eventually max out your line of energy credit. Your body stops metabolizing fat for energy, or your adrenal glands announce that you have gone to the well once too often and you encounter what's known as "adrenal insufficiency." You wind up energetically broke, overweight, and perhaps suffering from symptoms of chronic fatigue or some other serious illness. In the end, the metaphor of borrowing from a bank without paying back the loan may be too benign; it might be more accurate to compare this kind of dietary behavior to borrowing money from the Mob. If you don't pay back your energetic debt, your body may respond by sending out hit men to cripple your liver, kidneys, or intestinal tract!

THE ZONE

After low-cal, high-protein, and low-fat diets destabilized our blood sugar levels—exacerbated by coffee, grazing, and other forms of dietary instability—someone finally came up with a balanced diet that worked better than most of what had preceded it. In his book *The Zone,* Barry Sears proposed a regimen of 40 percent carbs, 30 percent protein, and 30 percent fat. Instead of changing the protein, fats, and carbs with the seasons as nature does, however, he doled them out equally all year long. This is still an improvement over eating an *un*balanced regimen all year round, as the other diets recommend.

Sears goes further, however, and restricts carbohydrate intake to low-glycemic carbs, meaning those that break down in the digestive tract most slowly and provide the longest-lasting fuel. That leaves out many perfectly good foods, including carrots, apples, potatoes, raisins, lima beans, pasta, and rice, all of which have either medium or high glycemic levels and burn more quickly than the low-glycemic carbs. Any diet that restricts such basic and healthful foods is unlikely to satisfy people for very long. As your hand reaches out for that beautiful Golden Delicious apple at a roadside farm market, you have to stop yourself and say, "Nope—burns too fast!" After 4 or 5 years of not eating high-glycemic carbs, moreover, you may well lose the ability to metabolize these foods at all. Quite frankly, no one knows the long-term effects of eating only low-glycemic-index foods, but the restrictive nature of this diet has already turned many away from it simply because, once again, it is too difficult to maintain.

The Zone is a great step in the right direction, seeking nature's balance of proteins, fats, and carbohydrates, but on a fixed, year-round basis rather than a seasonally adjusted one. This diet will certainly solve some of the problems generated by the blood sugar wars of the preceding decades, but it falls somewhat short of promoting a complete cycle of healthy eating.

CANDIDA, CHRONIC FATIGUE, AND EPSTEIN-BARR VIRUS

Undigested sugars and other indigestible foods that ferment in the intestine create the perfect breeding ground for candida, a yeast infection that was especially prevalent during the 1980s. Candida diets were created to eliminate sugar, dairy, fruit, wheat, and eggs in the hope of alleviating digestive stress and slowing fermentation. The candida would settle down until you had your first doughnut; then it would surge again, and fatigue and bloating would set in.

Around this time, large numbers of people were reporting symptoms of debilitating fatigue that could not readily be assigned to any known illness. This was a frustrating development for both physicians and their patients, since without knowing the cause, doctors could prescribe no clear remedy. Hundreds of articles were written about this mysterious disease, eventually labeled chronic fatigue syndrome (CFS), for which no effective cure was ever found. Some blamed it on a virus called Epstein-Barr, which again had no effective cure; not everyone who complained of CFS tested positive for Epstein-Barr, however, and confusion about the causes of these conditions abounded. What chronic fatigue, Epstein-Barr, and candida did have in common were fatigue and digestive distress. To solve the digestive distress, the best-selling book *Fit for Life* appeared, introducing a revolutionary new diet known as "food combining."

Based on the premise that different kinds of food are digested in different areas of the body, advocates of food combining recommended that exacting attention be paid to precisely what groups of food are consumed in concert. By eating at one sitting only those foods digested in the same part of the alimentary canal, this theory goes, one can relieve stress on the digestive system. Since proteins are digested primarily in the stomach and starches or carbohydrates are digested in the small intestine, they should not be eaten together. Removing stress from the digestive system not only aids digestion and avoids the problems caused by undigested food, it prevents the release of free radicals, the proliferation of candida yeast infections, and other toxins in the system.

By separating foods that are digested in different parts of the body, food combining also sought to relieve some of the many digestive disorders beginning to manifest in America, such as excess stomach acid, chronic indigestion, bloating, and gas. Unfortunately, food combining is very restrictive and somewhat unnatural in two ways. Certain common meals become anathema—for instance, eggs (protein) cannot be eaten together with potatoes or even a slice of toast (both starches); milk (protein) cannot be put on corn flakes (carbohydrate); meat or fish can no longer be combined with baked potatoes or rice. Besides this, all fruit must be eaten alone, never with a meal or even as dessert, and you must wait at least 20 to 30 minutes before eating anything else after having a piece of fruit. Although this diet worked to relieve some digestive symptoms and discomforts, it never addressed the underlying cause of the problem. As soon as you stop food combining, the symptoms come right back. This system of eating is a great medicinal tool, but you should not allow it to stop you short of your goal. In the end, combining led to eating smaller meals a few hours apart so that dieters could get in a wider variety of foods—a tactic that, if prolonged, like grazing, disrupted natural levels of blood sugar in the body.

COMING FULL CIRCLE

As we have seen already, the major drawback most people experienced with the high-protein diet was a lack of energy. So when Dr. Atkins recently reprised his version of this diet—27 years after his first book appeared—he allowed dieters to add more fat to their meals. He claimed that this would produce higher levels of conjugated linoleic acid, or CLA, "the only fatty acid to consistently, unequivocally inhibit cancer in lab rats." Since CLA appears abundantly in animal fat and red meat and has stronger antioxidant capabilities than beta carotene or vitamin E, Dr. Atkins recommends having steak every day if you like it (and can afford it).

Once again, such a diet may have short-term beneficial effects on dieters because of the introduction of a vast new source of nutrition to the body. But without a compensatory cleansing diet on the heels of such excess, as nature provides by following the high-protein, high-fat diet of winter with the low-fat cleansing regimen of spring, it can quickly get out of hand. Besides, excessive amounts of red meat have been proven to significantly increase the risk of colon cancer. Consuming so much protein just has too many potentially deleterious health effects to make this diet desirable. And there is another drawback in the form of a 95-page *Carbohydrate Gram Counter* that Atkins published as a companion piece. With only 20 grams of carbs allowed daily—about the equivalent of a small bowl of cereal—readers need to know exactly how many grams are in each bite. The very necessity for such a book underlines the main reason people will not stick with this diet for very long—it goes against the grain of human nature.

And so in the proliferation of fad diets over the decades, we have seen a cycle of sorts. This cycle, unfortunately, is not tied to nature but to an artificial attempt to address symptoms of overeating while ignoring the causes. In the following chapter, we will see how each of the three basic diets we have examined here fits into in the cycle of nature, satisfying our needs for proteins and carbohydrates, fats and sugars, without ever creating a deficiency that leads to food craving and overweight.

THE DIET-GO-ROUND

LOW-CALORIE DIETS

Diets began by limiting the number of calories consumed in a day. But restricting calories depleted energy, so people craved high-calorie fat and sugar as energizing emergency fuel.

LOW-FAT DIETS

High-calorie fats were targeted. Restricting fat left people hungry, however, and they again craved more fats and sugars.

FAKE FAT

Synthetic low-cal fats were invented. People could now replace butter with margarine, but without calories it didn't deliver the energy and satisfaction people needed. They still craved real fat and sugar.

THE DIET GO-ROUND

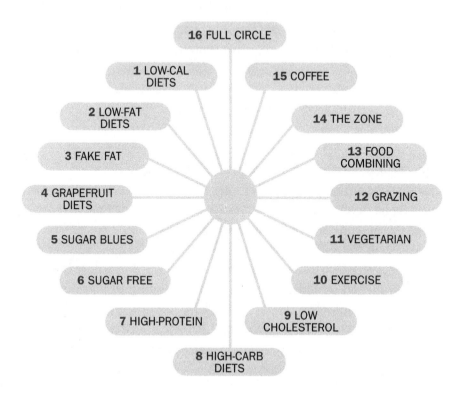

16 FULL CIRCLE

1 LOW-CAL DIETS

15 COFFEE

2 LOW-FAT DIETS

14 THE ZONE

3 FAKE FAT

13 FOOD COMBINING

4 GRAPEFRUIT DIETS

12 GRAZING

5 SUGAR BLUES

11 VEGETARIAN

6 SUGAR FREE

10 EXERCISE

7 HIGH-PROTEIN

9 LOW CHOLESTEROL

8 HIGH-CARB DIETS

GRAPEFRUIT DIETS

Banking on the antioxidant and fat-emulsifying properties of grapefruit, dieters could eat real fat again, as long as they ate a grapefruit first. But even grapefruits were no match for the high-fat American diet.

SUGAR BLUES

The more America restricted fat in any way to lose weight, the more the body rebounded by storing fat, and craving and bingeing on fats and sugars. Sugar was now to blame!

SUGAR FREE

High-calorie sugars were replaced with no-calorie synthetic sweeteners. The mind was happy but the body was starving as diet drinks replaced meals. People eventually binged on excess calories from other sources, such as protein.

HIGH-PROTEIN DIETS

The new diet let people eat all the protein they wanted without noticing the restriction of carbs and sugar. Energy came from fat stores and dieters lost weight. But without carbs, they soon experienced low energy and craved and binged on carbs.

HIGH-CARB DIETS

Carb-craving America was ripe for high-carb diets. You could now lose weight and eat up to 80 percent carbs—but they had to be slow-burning, complex carbs. Fast-paced America was addicted to fast energy, however, and high-carb diets soon became high-sugar diets.

LOW CHOLESTEROL

The combination of sugar, fat, and stress raised cholesterol to dangerous levels. The solution: Reemphasize complex carbs and reduce all animal fats. Once again, dieters felt restricted and began craving and bingeing on fats and sugars.

EXERCISE

Diets weren't working, so exercise became the cholesterol cure-all. It worked for a time, but people didn't like to "work out." Within 25 years, no more than 20 percent of Americans would do it regularly.

VEGETARIANISM

With heart disease and cancers on the rise, red meat was targeted. Vegetarianism came into fashion but was rarely followed correctly. People lived on pasta and bread, and blood sugars and energy levels went out of control.

GRAZING

High-carb diets were causing energy and blood sugar problems. If you ate every 2 hours, energy was propped up and fast-paced America could keep speeding. Fatigue became chronic fatigue, however, with depression and anxiety to follow.

FOOD COMBINING

By eating fats, proteins, and carbs separately, digestion improved and a host of digestive, energy, and weight problems were helped temporarily. But the rules for what you could eat together led to more frequent small meals. People eventually slipped back to their old ways and old problems.

THE ZONE

Aimed at fixing blood sugar levels, this diet balanced intake of proteins, fats, and carbs. It worked, but again restricted certain kinds of carbs, so it didn't last, and America was again craving emergency fuel.

COFFEE TO THE RESCUE

Exhausted and with a million things to do, America turned to legal stimulants like coffee for energy. But borrowed energy must be paid back, and many are still living in debt.

FULL CIRCLE

Frustrated, America is turning to new crash diets and a wave of high-protein diets. It is time to break this man-made cycle with the simplicity of nature's own 3-Season Diet. If you let nature feed you, you will not starve or crave anything.

CHAPTER 3

Converting Food to Energy: Medical and Historical Patterns

T O UNDERSTAND THE DAMAGE done to our systems by fad diets, fast food, and processed food, and to appreciate the need for a 3-Season Diet that gives us all of nature's nutrients in proper proportion over the course of a year, we have to take a brief look at how the body converts food to energy—the basic technology that keeps us alive on a daily basis.

We derive most of our energy from the fat, carbohydrates, and sugar in food, each of which the body metabolizes at different rates. By far, fat provides the slowest-burning, most consistent form of energy for the long haul. When our bodies are unstressed and metabolizing food properly, 42 percent of our total calories come from fat, more than from any other source. Carbohydrates provide somewhat faster-burning energy, however, which is why some athletes preparing for endurance events like the marathon practice "carbo-loading" beforehand, so that they will have quick access to fairly high levels of energy. Soft drinks, apples, bananas, vegetables, legumes, bread, pasta, even chocolate bars are all loaded with carbohydrates, although some forms are more beneficial than others. All carbohydrates are essentially composed of chains of simple sugars; "complex" carbohydrates, or polysaccharides, such as pasta, are made up of longer chains of sugars and burn more slowly and steadily than the simple, short-chain carbs found in potato or corn chips. (Some nutritionists complain that pasta is itself a processed food because the semolina is a processed form of wheat; yet people of many nations around the Mediterranean rim, not to mention China and the Far East, have lived healthy lives eating noodles for thousands of years.)

Simple sugar burns fastest of all and gives us the energy we need to handle the immediate stress of fight-or-flight situations. Unlike fat, which is metabolized slowly in the small intestine, sugar is metabolized in the mouth and stomach first, then the small intestine, so its energy is unleashed much more rapidly. Although sugar provides immediate energy—the so-called sugar rush of a sweetened soft drink or a candy bar—its burst of power is inevitably followed by a letdown, making it an extremely unreliable source of energy over long periods of time.

Throughout its evolutionary history, the human body burned primarily fat, reserving sugar stores for those emergency situations that required a quick, turbocharged burst of energy, like fighting an enemy or fleeing from a forest fire or a deadly animal. In tropical climates where human life is widely believed to have first emerged and developed, our earliest ancestors probably survived comfortably on a diet rich in carbohydrates from fruits and vegetation, along with occasional fats from foods such as fruits, fish, coconuts, avocados, and nuts readily available according to the season. In that essentially summertime climate, a predominantly carbohydrate diet was needed to cool and energize the body for the long hot days. The summer diet did not spike blood sugar levels because a sufficient supply of fats such as coconuts burned slowly and provided a baseline of steady energy, while sugars provided short bursts of intense energy in emergencies. Fats are naturally restricted in the spring as nature's harvest provides a low-fat, low-mucus diet of sprouts, leafy greens, berries, and roots. These fat-free foods force the body to burn its own fat for baseline energy. Fat is also where the body naturally stores toxins, so that a spring cleaning does happen in nature as we are forced to burn fat for fuel and toxins are released into the bloodstream to be eliminated.

But this kind of primal diet required such a large quantity of fruits, vegetables, and fiber that even a small growth in population forced people out of the proverbial Garden of Eden. Over time, much of humanity migrated to colder climates—which at the end of the last Ice Age would have been no farther north than lower Europe. These early humans, whose food supply was anything but regular and dependable, adapted to eating large meals at one sitting and living on that fuel for long periods. The human body learned to burn fat as a baseline energy supply and carbohydrates primarily for high energy, and to store sugar for emergencies. And so our ancestors came to rely on food sources rich in lipids (animal and vegetable fats), which gave them the ability to make energy last for days before they needed another meal. The protein in these winter meals gave them structural strength, and the fat gave them energy.

I once watched a documentary film about tigers in which the female tiger killed a wildebeest and fed her entire family with it. The narrator explained that she would not start hunting again for a week. Although carnivores have much quicker digestive systems than we do, we have lost the ability to make our food last over such a long haul. Many of us can't go even two hours without another meal. This is partly the result of the stressful ways we live our lives and our increasing need for emergency fuel, and partly due to the ready availability of snack food and junk food around the clock. Unfortunately, this way of eating will never balance our weight or provide us with adequate energy.

In survival scenarios such as prolonged hunger or extreme stress, the body reverses the age-old paradigm of burning fat and storing sugar for emergencies; it will instinctively store fat and burn sugar and, to a lesser extent, carbohydrates. Fat is the nutritional equivalent of gold under the mattress during a depression. Just as people caught in a financial crunch will sell off their least valuable possessions first to raise money, hanging on to gold or currency as long as they can, in emergencies your body wants to hold on to fat until the last possible moment because fat represents the most reliable source of energy.

In many popular starvation or deprivation diets, as we have seen, proteins will also be metabolized for energy. Although this is a more complicated process for the body, metabolizing protein represents a severe deprivation that is often triggered in those popular fad diets to burn body mass. This is risky business, because it has many complications regarding health and usually leads to uncontrollable rebound binge eating. In these deprivation diets, the body's metabolism is manipulated in such a way that stored fats are typically called on for immediate energy supply. If fats are not burned in combination with carbs to make energy, the body becomes more acidic than normal, because fat burning creates acid waste products that change the pH of the body to a bit more acid than alkaline. Just like the damaging effects of acid rain on the environment, burning too much fat and the attendant acid imbalance accelerates the degenerative processes in the body. In optimum health, the body is primarily alkaline in balance rather than acid; and our bodies function best when about 70 percent of our diet is alkaline.

A slow, steady pace to life leads naturally to eating foods that provide slow- and steady-burning energy, storing the proper amount of fat to be burned for fuel as needed throughout the long workday. During the agricultural era, the big meal of the day was usually the midday meal, replenishing stores burnt up in the heavy labor of the morning and fueling the brain and nervous system for the rest of the day. By evening, fat and calories from that big meal had been pretty much worked off, and a light supper was easily digested during the night.

Many of our misperceptions about the role of fat and other foods in our diet began to take shape, however, during more than a century of monumental change in Western life. Once the onset of the Industrial Revolution in the mid-18th century began a gradual shift away from the traditional meal schedule associated with agricultural life, we began to lose touch with the natural cycle of consuming food and burning energy. As more people worked in factories and offices, often between increasingly long commutes, lunch became an inconvenience that interrupted the limited amount of time in the workday. Modern workers chose to run errands, work through lunch, or even exercise at lunchtime, thinking that they were being virtuous and efficient by "sacrificing" their free time. The body was increasingly forced to wait until evening for its big meal, when the family was home from work and school. But the body does not digest food as efficiently at the end of the day, when its energy is winding down and getting ready for sleep, and so digestion was compromised. It's not surprising that the 20th century has been awash in ever more potent remedies for indigestion and acid stomach upset.

True to its name, fast food accelerated the change in ancient patterns of eating. Burgers, hot dogs, pizza, fries, and milk shakes provide large amounts of fat, carbohydrates, and sugar rather cheaply compared to, say, a well-balanced home-cooked or restaurant meal, but they do so at a price that far outweighs the financial savings. Because this food is highly processed and cooked so quickly, it is largely indigestible. The longer fatty food such as meat is cooked, the more digestible it becomes. Burgers, deep-fried chicken and potatoes that are prepared in a matter of minutes at a fast-food restaurant or even in a home microwave are much harder for the body to digest than, say, a braised lamb shank cooked for hours in its own juices. Besides, the kind of meal that takes longer to prepare is usually eaten slowly around a dinner table rather than around a steering wheel on the way home. The lamb shank may have as many calories as the burger, yet the body will metabolize it more efficiently and so less of it will be stored as fat. Have you ever found a french-fried potato that fell behind a garbage can or car seat and was left there for months? It may be a little harder and drier but it's usually still recognizable. A piece of raw meat or fruit exposed that long would have virtually disappeared, consumed by bacteria. But deep-frying will preserve that scrap of potato for posterity, protecting it not only from bacteria in the air but also from the enzymes and bacteria in your digestive tract.

Processing, which strips crucial foods such as nuts and grains of their essential fatty oils and nutrients, began long before the first McDonald's appeared on the American landscape. Back in the 1950s, milk was homogenized for our convenience, processing it in such a way that the cream no longer separated; its shelf life was extended, but it became far less digestible as a result. Nutritionists who insist that dairy products are bad for us are right when they refer to today's milk and milk products. Although milk does have valuable nutrients, it was meant to be drunk in small amounts in certain seasons—whole, nonhomogenized, and even nonpasteurized, never ice-cold, and certainly not loaded with the residue of growth hormones and antibiotics fed to cows. It is true that some ethnic groups do not have the enzymes to digest milk, but it is also true that today's milk is extremely hard to digest.

High amounts of refined sugar in shakes and sodas, and the simple-carbohydrate sugars of hamburger buns and fries provide the emergency fuel many people crave to handle growing levels of stress. Unfortunately, this food also contains excessive amounts of fat and carbohydrate, which are stored as fat because the body is unable to metabolize them fast enough. Perhaps the most disastrous side effect of this constant diet of sugars and carbs is that over time our bodies have lost their innate ability to metabolize fat for fuel. Why burn fat when we can more easily get it from sugar and simple carbohydrates like bread and chips? So even when we ate a properly balanced meal at home in leisure, the body no longer processed the food in the traditional way. As we will see, the 3-Season Diet ensures that the body can burn fat by resetting its ability to do so with a low-fat spring harvest that moves the body into fat metabolism. This guarantees that blood sugars remain stable during the high-sugar-and-carb harvest of summer. Following the active months of summer, the body will welcome the fall harvest of high-nutrient foods rich in proteins and fats that are needed to rebuild and restore those reserves for winter. The diet comes full circle in spring, when any excess of these heavy winter foods is cleansed by the spring harvest.

If we look at two social groups who may eat fast food most often today, some illuminating patterns emerge. People in the lower economic echelons eat fast food of necessity because it does provide most of the essential nutrients for life very inexpensively. It's hard to beat a whole meal with protein, carbs, sugars, and fats for under five dollars. Sadly, since these fast-food meals are overloaded with fats and are indigestible to boot, obesity and hypertension levels have risen even faster among the working poor in this country than among other segments of the population.

Another group that accounts for a large proportion of fast-food sales is teenagers. Despite the boundless energy that allows young people to burn off overly fatty and processed foods, obesity is rising most rapidly among this age group. Part of the reason is that television, the computer, and the automobile have rendered youthful lives far less active than they once were, countering teens' innate ability to burn calories at a prodigious rate.

Both teenagers and the working classes are drawn to fast food for other reasons. Because this food provides a feeling of comfort, satiety, and quick energy—however illusory or short lived—it has a special appeal for people whose lives are not especially easy or trouble-free in other ways. If you have to take three buses to get to work and scramble each month to pay the rent, or are struggling mightily with acne, schoolwork, and raging hormones, then a greasy burger and salty fries, or a slice of pizza and a giant Coke may be the emotional highlight of your day. This is especially true if you skipped lunch at school because "nobody likes the junk they serve you." The people at Mcdonald's know exactly what they are talking about when they call their fast-food specials aimed at children "Happy Meals."

To make things harder all around, in the last few decades families have been finding it increasingly necessary for both parents to enter the workforce. The ideal of equal rights for women quickly devolved into the concept of the superwoman—an ordinary human being who is expected to complete her education and start her career while still shouldering most of the traditional burden of caring for the children. Maneuvering in an increasingly competitive workplace and attempting to brush off feelings of guilt at not being home with the kids, women are nonetheless supposed to maintain the unrealistic weight profile that was foisted on them by Madison Avenue and the fashion industry. When such stressors were added to a diet that already craved emergency fuel in the form of sugars and carbs, and at a time of abundant and readily available food, the body began to store fat from the excess of fats and carbs as never before.

THE INDIGESTION FACTOR

Apart from the discomfort of an upset stomach due to "acid indigestion," what's so dangerous about weakened or dysfunctional digestion? For one thing, when food is not completely digested by the intestines, it tends to break down partially and remain there, coating the intestinal tract with mucus. This is exacerbated by the kinds of foods we now eat. The *American Journal of Public Health* reports that only 9 percent of Americans eat the recommended number of servings of fruits and vegetables each day, 45 percent do not eat any fruit or drink any fruit juice, and 22 percent do not eat any vegetables at all. The foods we eat the most—bread, pasta, dairy products, and meat—are all highly mucus producing. This mucus gums up the workings of the intestines like tar in a dirty air filter; the body cannot absorb the muck, and what nutrients do get though it into the bloodstream are somewhat tainted. (Nutritionists say that our diet should be 70 percent alkaline because alkaline foods remove mucus and balance the standard American high-acid diet.) While the resulting impurities are being transported in the blood and lymph, they are oxidized, like rust, and by the time they reach the liver they have been converted into free radicals that damage the liver and compromise its ability to cleanse the blood and manufacture nutrients.

It is the job of the lymphatic system, part of the body's waste-removal mechanism, to flush free radicals (which are also produced by stress) and other impurities out of the body. But before the free radicals can be removed, they may attach themselves to fat cells that are also on their way to the liver and create lipid peroxides, which we know to generate the high cholesterol levels that lead to arterial plaque and ultimately heart disease. (Lipid peroxides are toxic products formed by the oxidation of fats, usually unsaturated fatty acids. Composed of unstable molecules, they scavenge other unsuspecting lipids and damage them through oxidation.) Cholesterol levels have far less to do with the amount of fat ingested than with the relative indigestibility of the food taken in and the resultant levels of stress that produce free radicals.

Although a certain amount of mucus production is natural in the winter, when winter foods help keep us from drying out, too many mucus-producing foods year round can become a perfect breeding ground for yeast, bad bacteria, and parasites. That makes it all the more important to change our diet as we go into the spring in ways I will show you, to take advantage of the low-fat, low-mucus, and high-alkaline foods that nature provides. The extent to which you get dried out in the winter because you did not eat a high-protein, high-fat diet consisting of warm and oily foods is to the extent to which you will produce excess mucus in the spring. It may manifest as a spring cold, cough, allergy, asthma, or the proliferation of yeast in the intestines, as the mucus membranes in the intestines will also produce excess mucus.

The excessive amounts of fat found in a typically greasy fast-food burger or a slab of pizza with pepperoni not only add more mucus, but also make the body work harder to break down all that fat to get to the protein and carbohydrates. Food that is incompletely broken down and remains in the digestive tract also putrefies, ferments, promotes bloating, and creates a fertile breeding ground for candida, parasites, and destructive bacteria. This has led to a series of energy-related disorders including chronic fatigue, Epstein-Barr syndrome, fibromyalgia, and a mushrooming incidence of anxiety and depression. All of these factors in turn increase stress on the digestive system and vital organs, producing more free radicals in a potentially debilitating cycle.

Just as the energy rush engendered by sugars and simple carbs quickly wears off and leads to an energy crash later in the day, relying for energy on the kinds of foods that our bodies have such difficulty digesting properly can, over the years, set us up for a large-scale reckoning in the form of chronic fatigue, anxiety, and depression. These chronic conditions make it all the more difficult to live the life of calm, steady vitality that would make the whole idea of fast food seem absurd and undesirable in the first place.

WHY WE NEED ALL THE BASIC FORMS OF NUTRIENTS

One key reason the fad diets of the past century have been so unsuccessful and even harmful is that, as I've pointed out, they insist on restricting one form of food or another. The problem with restricting basic kinds of nutrients from the diet is that our bodies are programmed to make use of all of them. Proteins, carbohydrates, fats, and sugars each serve a distinct purpose, and trying to do without one group for the mere expedient of losing weight is just another example of paddling against the current. Take protein, for example, which is found in meat, fish, dairy, legumes, nuts, seeds, and grains. The nutritionists who insist that we need only a tiny amount of protein overlook the wide range of crucial functions protein performs in the body. It is the body's principal source of enzymes and hormones and is needed for building the musculoskeletal system (muscles, bones, hair, nails, and teeth), as well as for certain aspects of blood and for the growth and maintenance of all tissues. Protein also contains essential amino acids, which are not made by the body and must be gotten from food. Animal proteins have all 22 essential amino acids in them, as do certain combinations of foods, such as rice and beans. Some diets seek to limit protein intake, however, because many of the foods that contain protein, especially animal protein, also contain fat. And fat is bad for us, right? Let's take a closer look.

Fat has suffered from perhaps the worst press of any vital nutritional substance known to humanity, but despite what you may have read, we all need a certain amount of fat in our diets. As we have seen, the underlying premise of almost every diet to have emerged in the last 50 years is that fat is somehow bad for us, an assumption based on the simple observation that people become overweight and obese by storing more fat than their bodies can metabolize. The real problem, however, lies in the way the body is artificially stimulated by many diets to burn fat and then soon after store it, rather than burn it steadily as it ought to. Moreover, the body craves fat for a reason: Besides serving as our most reliable fuel source, fat also makes hormones and contributes to vital cell processes. Fatty oils in the body act as transportation systems for carrying the fat-soluble vitamins A, D, E, and K and certain minerals to the tissues and vital organs, not to mention lubricating the skin and hair. If you look at the body of a newborn baby next to that of an 80-year-old, you will see a startling difference: clear, lustrous, wrinkle-free skin that is soft and resilient to the touch, compared to dried out, nonflexible, and cracking skin, flaking scalp, and brittle hair. The difference is oil.

The triglycerides in fat hold our internal organs in position, insulate the body against cold, suppress gastric secretions, and serve another, perhaps even more significant, function. Lipids (fats) themselves have no taste, but their chemical structure enables them to trap pleasurable flavors. The oil in tomato sauce lets it cling not only to your spaghetti but to your taste buds as well. The fat component is responsible for your feeling of satisfaction after a meal, a sensation that springs in part from the fact that fats and oils leave the stomach more slowly than proteins and carbs after a meal, and this retards hunger. Vegetable oils and most fish also contain essential fatty acids that are needed by the body to keep cholesterol levels down. Eskimos, who live in a climate of nearly constant winter and eat a diet almost totally lacking in vegetables, have an extremely low incidence of heart disease because their diet is also high in insulating and warm marine lipids containing essential fatty acids (EFAs—so-called omega-3 and omega-6 oils). Far from causing obesity, in fact, the proper amount of fat in the diet actually helps prevent both the overeating that promotes weight gain and the cholesterol that leads to heart disease.

The healthful Mediterranean Diet mentioned earlier relies heavily on the use of oils made from seeds and nuts and to a lesser extent on fish oils. Walnut, canola, safflower, and flaxseed oil are unsaturated, so they do not raise blood levels of cholesterol and are rich in alpha-linolenic acid, an omega-3 fatty acid found only in plants and essential to human health. Together with the oil in fish—which contains the omega-3 unsaturated fatty acids known as eicosapentaenoic acid, or EPA, and docosahexaenoic acid, or DHA—these oils have been shown to reduce the risk of blood clotting, abnormal heart rhythms, and the creation of arterial plaque. Surprisingly, fats provide more than twice the energy, gram for gram, of carbohydrates, the more generally accepted source of energy. Up to two-thirds of the total energy of the cells may be supplied by fats rather than carbohydrates. Because of its high density and slow-burning nature, another primary function of fat is to store energy in its cells. If we eat more food than we need, however, unused proteins and carbohydrates will also be stored in the fat cells, leading to weight gain and reducing energy levels.

Another misconception about fat is making Americans fatter by the day. According to Dr. Alice H. Lichtenstein, a professor of nutrition at Tufts University in Boston, "People assumed that if a food had no fat, they could eat as much of it as they wanted. But many low-fat and fat-free products have nearly as many calories as their full-fat versions. Reducing fat alone is no guarantee of weight loss. You must cut calories or increase physical activity." In fact, "fat-free," "reduced fat," and "non-fat" products often have *more* calories than their "regular" counterparts. The new National Heart, Lung, and Blood Institute Obesity Guidelines urge you to compare calories. A fat-free fig cookie has 70 calories, but a regular one has only 50, while a half-cup of nonfat ice cream or frozen yogurt yields 10 calories more than the regular version.

The revival of high-protein diets in recent years is largely a response to the fact that, as I pointed out in chapter 2, low-fat diets led to bingeing on carbohydrates. Dr. Margo Denke, an associate professor of medicine and endocrinology at the University of Texas Southwestern Medical Center in Dallas, agrees and warns against avoiding fat at the cost of adding calories: "No matter what anyone tells you, it's calories that count. Carefully controlled metabolic studies show that it doesn't matter where extra calories come from. Eat more calories than you expend and you'll gain weight." And that is just what Americans have been doing: gaining weight on fat-free and low-fat foods consumed without regard to their caloric content. Instead of replacing some of the less desirable high-fat foods like dairy and red meat with nutrient-rich but low-calorie fruits and vegetables, the experts lament, dieters are filling up on "low-fat" foods loaded with added sugars and refined starches that have little to offer nutritionally besides calories.

"In making food choices, we must learn to eat foods that are nutritionally robust—fruits, vegetables, legumes," says Dr. Robert H. Eckel, chairman of the American Heart Association's nutrition committee and professor of medicine and physiology at the University of Colorado. "There is strong evidence that these kinds of foods help to reduce disease, not just heart disease but also cancer, diabetes, hypertension, and obesity."

SUGAR, SUGAR

Next to fat, the most maligned nutrient may well be sugar, or small-chain carbohydrates. The simplest kinds of carbohydrates, which we commonly call sugar, are monosaccharides and disaccharides, meaning they are made of either one or two sugars. The most common monosaccharide by far is glucose, which requires no alterations to be absorbed and utilized by the body and so is responsible for most of the energy we receive. Glucose is also responsible for the functional integrity of the nervous system and is the sole source of energy in the brain. Fructose, which is found in fruit, and galactose, or milk sugar, are two other common monosaccharides. The two most common disaccharides are sucrose, a combination of glucose and fructose; and lactose, a combination of glucose and galactose. All these mono- and disaccharides are primarily stored in the liver and muscles as glycogen, to be used as energy. Glycogen is a very large molecule called a polysaccharide, because it is a long chain of simple sugars. Starch is a polysaccharide found in grains, roots, vegetables, and legumes. The hallmark of a starch is that it is encased in the plant cell by cellulose. Starches are insoluble in cold water and must be cooked to release the starch from its cellulose or fibrous wall. Cooking starches softens the cellulose, and as the cell wall ruptures the starch is ready to be processed by the body as energy. Cellulose is also a polysaccharide, but we do not have the enzymes needed to digest it. It acts as fiber or bulk for our intestines and stimulates peristalsis, which promotes regular bowel movements. Cellulose is found in fruit, stalks, and leaves and the outer covering of grains, nuts, seeds, and legumes.

We need sugar for a variety of functions, although the form in which we get our sugar is crucial. All fruits and most vegetables contain some sugar, called fructose in fruit, and glucose in vegetables and grains. The "glycemic index" touted by certain diets measures the relative rate of release of fructose or glucose by most fruits, vegetables, legumes, and grains. Sucrose is the most abundant sugar in plants, but once it has been refined from, say, sugar cane or beets, it has no nutrients; known as table sugar, it should be avoided in its refined form. Many unrefined forms of sugar make acceptable sweeteners, however, such as Sucanat and other forms of dried sugar cane.

CARBOHYDRATES AND THE SEROTONIN SOLUTION

The nutrients perhaps most widely accepted as being healthful and necessary to good nutrition are carbohydrates. Carbs are found in fruits, vegetables, legumes, breads, cereals, potatoes and other starches, syrups, dairy products, and grains. Some diet experts, however, insist that because many grains are processed to make staple foods such as pasta and bread, they are an undesirable form of carbohydrate for many people. It's true that certain "simple" carbohydrates, like those found in most varieties of chips and many candies, can cause weight gain and should be avoided, but more complex carbs do not create any such problems. And we need them because we derive most of our basic energy, particularly for our brains, from the glucose in carbs. When high-protein diets minimize the need for more than a very small level of carbohydrate intake, they overlook the role of carbs in providing the massive amounts of energy our central nervous system needs to function smoothly throughout the day. As we have seen, restricting the amount of carbs in the diet can lead to low energy and wildly fluctuating blood sugar levels.

In the early 1980s, researchers discovered a link between serotonin and eating disorders that appeared to underline the problems associated with a high-protein diet. Serotonin is a neurotransmitter that regulates mood by producing a sense of well-being, and is responsible for handling stress. Reduced levels of serotonin in the brain can lead to depression and, in extreme cases, to aggressive behaviors, obsessive compulsive disorder, violence, and suicide. Studies at the Clinical Research Center at MIT conducted by Richard and Judith Wurtmann, and explained in Judith Wurtmann's book *The Serotonin Solution,* found that sweet and starchy foods, from doughnuts to tortillas, increase levels of serotonin in the brain. For this reason, these forms of carbohydrates can be considered psychoactive.

The Wurtmanns theorized that digested carbohydrates convert to the sugars of which they are composed, and this stimulates the pancreas to release insulin. In turn, insulin raises the level in the brain of tryptophan, an amino acid linked to serotonin production. Since the release of serotonin produces an overall sense of well-being in brain and body, when overweight people binge on carbs such as bread, pizza, and fries, they are self-medicating to elevate their mood. The Wurtmann's studies of obese women, for instance, revealed that eating a snack high in carbohydrates improved their mood and that much the same was true for premenstrual women and smokers trying to quit. The knowledge that they have just eaten more than they should may, however, result in feelings of guilt or low self-worth, which can lead to depression and the need for another mood lift via carbo-bingeing. The same researchers found that rats on high-protein diets binged excessively on carbs as soon as they came off the diet. Protein diets release numerous amino acids into the blood, and the excess aminos compete with tryptophan uptake by the brain, lowering levels of serotonin production and forcing the body into an emergency craving response. In this case, restricting one essential nutrient—carbohydrates—leads chemically to the need to binge on the restricted food. No matter how much weight you may lose at first from such a restrictive diet, you are laying the groundwork for gaining it all back in the end.

Now that we have seen the importance of each of nature's nutrients, and the dangers of restricting any of them unduly from the diet, let's take a look at how you can be assured of getting all these nutrients in the proportions that nature originally intended. Let's see what Nature's Meal Plan looks like on a year-round basis.

CHAPTER 4

The 3-Season Meal Plan

A S WE HAVE SEEN, the 3-Season Diet is derived from the three primary harvests: a light harvest in the spring; a fruit and vegetable harvest all summer; and a heavier, fall harvest of foods for the winter. Correspondingly, the diet emphasizes different qualities in each season—a low-fat, lower-calorie diet in spring; high-carb in summer; and high-protein and fat in winter. But this does not mean that carbs are avoided in winter or protein in the spring. Protein, fat, and carbs always have to be in the diet to some extent, but the proportions fluctuate as the seasons change. Spring calls for roughly 10 percent of your diet to come from fats, about 60 percent from carbs, and 30 percent from protein. In summer, carbs make up nearly 80 percent of the total harvest and should provide at least 60 to 70 percent of your diet, with the rest split about equally between protein and fat. And in winter, 40 percent of your food should be protein, 30 percent fat, and 30 percent carbs.

These percentages should not be measured with a calculator or gram counter, however. In nature the basic idea is to eat more proteins in winter, which should come quite naturally, as that's when you probably already prefer soups, grains, nuts, and meats. In the spring eat more salads, sprouts, greens, and berries, and in summer eat fruits and vegetables in copious amounts. Shopping from the grocery lists at the end of chapter 5 and in Appendix 3 will make this process simple, and soon you will instinctively know and desire a natural shift in your diet from one season to the next. Since protein, carbs, and fat can each be derived from a wide variety of food types, I'll explain some of the general characteristics of fruits, vegetables, grains, dairy, and meat, and then go on to a complete breakdown of the best foods to eat in each of the three seasons.

FRUITS

In the tropics where human life began, heat is abundant and fruits are harvested all year round. Made up mostly of carbohydrates, vitamins, and minerals with very little protein or fat content, they are still best eaten in summer, when their cooling influence acts as an antidote to the heat. The high levels of carbohydrates in fruit provide energy during the very active summer months with their long days and short nights. Today, sadly, many people cannot eat fruit as it doesn't satisfy their hunger or it wreaks havoc with their blood sugar levels, which have become fragile from faulty eating habits. As you will see with the 3-Season Diet Plan later in this chapter, nature took into consideration the high-sugar content of fruit by creating a low-fat harvest in the spring. The low-fat spring harvest annually resets the body's ability to metabolize fat as fuel, forcing the body to burn its own fat for energy. When the high-energy, high-carb summer harvest arrives, the body's baseline energy supply has already been set from the fat-burning of spring, preventing the high-sugar foods of summer from causing blood sugar highs and lows.

In a northern climate where no fruit occurs naturally in the winter, we need heavier foods to insulate and warm us against the cold—nuts, oils, and other sources of fat and protein. Some fruits grown in other parts of the world, however, have the same winter-balancing qualities of warmth, heaviness, and higher fat for insulation found in winter foods. Avocados and bananas are two fruits that prove this point; even though they are not harvested in Vermont in the winter, they are perfectly fine during the cold winter months. Other fruits are helpful in winter because of their sweet, sour, and heavy qualities, and they can be cooked to enhance their winter-balancing properties. Oranges harvested in Florida in the early winter, for example, are sweet, slightly sour, and heavy, with high water content—all ideal qualities for balancing winter. And avocados contains 25 percent fat, making them the highest-fat fruit in the world—a seemingly perfect winter fruit even if we think of it as a summer food. Avocados actually came from the tropics, and the original Mexican *aguacate*, its sister the *topa topa*, and hundreds of other varieties were all winter-maturing types. Nature seems to have understood perfectly how to keep us in balance simply by the wisdom of its harvest. (In the Glossary of Foods, (Appendix 1), each food will be explained in greater detail with its original harvest, nutritional qualities, and best season for eating.)

In the spring most fruits are not yet ripe or harvested, and so dried fruits are a better bet. In traditional farming communities, fruits were dried in the fall to be stored all winter and eaten in the spring when the harvest is sparse. The spring is also a great time to eat sprouts of any kind, because that is exactly what nature is doing–sprouting. Lentils, garbanzos, peas, limas, adzukis, alfalfa, clover, radish, and wheat berry beans fall off the stalk in the fall and lie on the ground all winter, until they begin to sprout in early spring. The deer are smart enough to thrive on them, and so should we be. Sprouts are loaded with vitamins, nutrients, and chlorophyll, a natural blood cleanser.

Because fresh fruit juices concentrate the cooling effects of fruit, they can be mixed with spices such as ginger, lemon juice, salt, cardamom, clove, and cinnamon to enhance their digestibility–particularly in the spring and winter when the cooling properties are not necessary. The same is true of very sweet fruits such as melons. Melons also don't mix well with other foods and are best taken alone, but can be flavored with salt and lemon juice to improve their digestibility. Sour fruits like lemons, pineapples, papayas, and cranberries digest well and are more easily taken with other foods. Most fruits easily mix with grains but not so well with vegetables.

VEGETABLES

Vegetables are generally harvested in the spring and summer, but 100 years ago our diet consisted of a higher percentage of root vegetables, typically harvested in the spring and fall. Most of the heavy, warming root vegetables are harvested in the fall, including beets, carrots, and potatoes, which are loaded with minerals and vitamins to combat the dryness of winter. Lighter veggies are harvested in the spring: sprouts of all kinds, leafy greens, green beans, asparagus, spinach, kale, Swiss chard, and mustard greens, all of which have just the antimucus and low-fat qualities you need in spring. Because the body holds on to more water in the spring, which can result in excess mucus production, nature offers relief with the harvest of mucus-breaking bitter roots such as onions, garlic, echinacea, golden seal, burdock root, chicory, and Oregon grape. We stopped chewing on roots about 100 years ago, but after the winter snows melt and plants are exposed, the deer chew on surface roots called rhizomes that are loaded with blood-purifying, liver-strengthening properties. Keep in mind that the deeper roots are what support the plant; if the rhizomes are eaten the plant continues to flourish. This is another way nature ensures our health and well-being—but we have stopped taking its advice.

During spring as the ground softens and plants push up out of the soil, our bodies soften by holding on to more water. The body rehydrates, and the excess fluids flush it of toxins. These toxins often head toward the liver to be processed, but if the bitter greens, roots, and rhizomes are not taken at this time the liver can get overwhelmed and inefficiently deal with the seasonal cleansing. One example of the curative powers of bitter roots shows up in recent research on chicory, a perennial plant that, like dandelion, has a deep spiraling taproot and grows wild in yards and by roadsides. Its young leaves and roots have traditionally been used for their diuretic and liver-protecting qualities. According to the *Journal of Ethnopharmacology,* researchers in Pakistan, where the plant has long been popular as a folk remedy for liver disease, have shown that extracts from chicory root inhibit oxidative degradation of DNA in liver tissue, a beneficial effect.

The extent to which you get dried out in the winter because you did not eat warm and oily foods is the extent to which you will produce mucus in excess in the spring. It may manifest as a spring cold, cough, allergy, asthma, or the proliferation of yeast in the intestines, as the mucous membranes in the intestines will also produce excess mucus. Nature will automatically prevent these fatiguing allergenic symptoms if only we eat what it harvests. Bitter greens and roots will scrape the mucus off the intestines and clean the blood while helping the liver do its big spring cleaning job. You have only to look about you to notice the abundance of bright green foliage lining the countryside in the spring. Those green seedlings, sprouts, and buds are extremely rich in chlorophyll. Chlorophyll acts as a fertilizer for good bacterial growth in the intestines. The natural spring harvest provides bitter roots to remove excess mucus from the heavy fare of winter and fertilizes good bacterial growth in the intestines to prevent the proliferation of yeast, parasites, and bad bacteria. Many of us see the dandelions that appear in our yards each spring as nuisance weeds to be rooted out, but they are there in such numbers for a reason. Pick the dandelion greens from your own backyard, wash them, and boil them in water with a little salt into a dandelion tea, eat them in salads, or sauté them lightly with a little oil and garlic.

The goal of the spring is to cleanse the excess fat and protein of a long, low-metabolic winter and to restimulate the body to burn fat as fuel throughout the spring and summer. This restimulation naturally detoxifies the proteins and extra carbs stored in the fat cells. Pungent vegetables like onions and chilies increase metabolism and digestive strength and help to burn off the excess protein and fat, while many of the natural diuretic vegetables such as mustard greens, parsley, celery, asparagus, cilantro, lettuce, and watercress work to remove the excess water that the body tends to hold on to in the spring. Although not always harvested in the spring, broccoli, potatoes, and carrots also help reduce excess water in the body.

In the summer, with the harvest of cucumbers, broccoli, cauliflower, zucchini, okra, bell peppers, tomatoes, peas, and celery, vegetables shift from cleansing and fat-free in nature to more nutritious, energy producing, and cooling. As more substantial vegetables are harvested, they provide us with greater energy to endure the longer days and higher energy demands of summer in natural harmony with the beginning of the summer fruit harvest. It's best to eat more raw vegetables in summer, and in the winter more cooked veggies. In the spring more salads and leafy greens, spiced to enhance digestibility, are called for.

GRAINS

Grains are all harvested in the fall to provide a high-protein, high-fat diet and an adequate carbohydrate energy base to make it through the long winter. All grains can, of course, be stored and last throughout the year and can be eaten at any time in moderation. In general, almost all grains are acceptable in winter because, although they are high in carbs, they also tend to be high in protein and essential fatty acids compared to fruits and vegetables. Some grains are more cooling than others, which makes them more appropriate for summer, including barley, oats, wheat, rice, and rye. In spring, you should avoid the glutenous grains such as wheat, and heavy grains like rice and moist oats. Although many grains have dry properties that are good for spring, this is not the best time of year to consume them.

Yeasted breads make gas and are more difficult to digest in the winter, and their sticky quality can exacerbate the spring environment that is already heavy and somewhat sticky. Yeast produces excess mucus in the intestines, which is particularly a problem in spring, the so-called allergy season, when the body is holding on to more water and tends to make more mucus. Toasting helps to decrease the mucus production, but in general you should eat less yeasted bread, especially wheat, especially in spring but also all year round. We eat so much wheat that we should try to minimize our intake. It was originally a grain for cold, dry climates, but we eat it everywhere. Wheat isn't bad in itself, but the glutens in wheat eaten in excess tend to gum up the digestive tract.

Dried grains like crackers are better in the spring when dry foods serve as an antidote to the wet nature of spring. In the winter cooked grains are heavier and warming, helping to combat the cold and dryness. Most people think of grains as a high-carb food, which they are. Yet the proportion of fat and protein in winter grains is much higher than the proportions found in the fruits and vegetables of summer. Unrefined grains are loaded with essential fatty acids and proteins, making them one of the plant kingdom's highest sources of essential fatty acids and protein, very close to beans and nuts, which are also harvested and eaten in the winter. Many traditional cultures still get most of their protein needs from grains.

LEGUMES

Beans that are harvested in the fall are considered legumes and should not be confused with vegetables such as green beans or string beans, which are spring harvested. Legumes produce gas because of the hard-to-digest hard fiber shell that protects the bean from rot and rancidity and allows it to last for years if need be. So even though logic might suggest that beans are good winter foods because they are harvested in the fall, they actually work even better in the spring and summer when their gas does not add to the drying effect of winter winds. They are best either when soaked and cooked very well or as sprouted beans, since those provide us with chlorophyll and energy.

THE BENEFITS OF SPROUTING

You can sprout almost any nut, seed, legume, or grain. Sprouting is the natural activity of germination that typically takes place in the spring. In this process the acid nut, grain, or seed becomes a more easily digested alkaline food. The process also releases proteins into more digestible amino acids; long-chain carbs are broken down into shorter chains, and fats into more easily absorbed fatty acids. Along with this, many more vitamins and minerals are released during the germination process. Enzymes necessary to digest the sprout are released and chlorophyll is manufactured in large quantities. The heaviness of a grain such as wheat is lightened as the gluten content in the wheat sprout or wheat grass is nullified. Sprouts are so naturally nutritious and cleansing as to be an absolute requirement for our spring diet.

RECIPE FOR SPROUTS IN THE SPRING

Place a large handful of sunflower seeds, mung beans, or whatever you are sprouting into a large glass jar with a screened or perforated top. Cover the seeds with three to four times as much water. Soak them for a few hours or overnight, then drain the water and rinse the beans. Put the jar on its side in a dark place for 1 to 3 days, rinsing and shaking the beans once or twice a day. Do not let the beans dry out. When they germinate and start to sprout, place the jar in indirect or intermittent direct sunlight and keep them moist. When the sprouts are green on the tips, they are ready to eat. Refrigerate them and eat them with meals, as snacks, or anytime you like.

When harvested, the bean is a high-protein food and very acid in nature. Just as acid disturbs the balance of life in many forests and streams, so acid foods in excess can create a harmful imbalance in the diet. Many nutritionists agree that only 30 percent of our diet should be acid and the rest should be alkaline, which is also predominant in our bodies. For this reason, many diet books recommend restricting breads, nuts, and meats because they are high in acid, and eating more vegetables and fruits, which are naturally alkaline. Without doubt our diet is heavily skewed to the acid side, and many experts agree that this high-acid diet is linked to many of our chronic health problems, from arthritis to allergies. Most of the acid foods are harvested in the fall for the winter, and most of the alkaline foods are harvested in the spring and summer. So by following the 3-Season Diet you will automatically balance your pH by getting most of the body-building high-protein, high-acid foods in the winter, making up about one-third of your diet, and most of the alkaline foods in the spring and summer, making up the other two-thirds. Once again nature has already addressed the issue of acid and alkaline foods as it changes its harvest with each season. A bean harvested in the fall, for instance, is an acid food, but if left to lie on the ground, it will sprout in the spring and become alkaline. So beans can be either well cooked in winter to build you up or sprouted in the spring to clean you out.

Mung beans and tofu (made from soybeans) are useful in the winter because of their high concentration of nutrients, as are most beans, provided you cook them long enough, spice them properly, and don't eat them in excess. You should soak the beans overnight and parboil them (bring the beans to a boil three or four times, each time replacing the water), which is also helpful to enhance their digestibility and their healthful effects, as I will explain in the part of this chapter dealing with winter diet.

PERFECT PROTEIN SOUP

This soup is very easy to digest and can be eaten all year long. You could live on it alone for quite some time if need be. I recommend it especially for anyone with digestive difficulties like gas, malabsorption of food, or chronic fatigue. This soup makes a great medicine to rebuild the body without digestive difficulties, and so is ideal for babies, women after giving birth, the elderly, or anyone in a weakened condition. Spicing beans with onions, *hing* (asafetida), cumin, fennel, cayenne, salt, pepper, and cardamom helps produce less gas.

INGREDIENTS

1 cup split yellow mung beans

2 cups white basmati rice

1 inch fresh gingerroot, chopped

1 small handful fresh cilantro leaves, chopped

2 tbs. ghee (clarified butter)

1 tsp. turmeric

1 tsp. coriander powder

1 tsp. cumin powder

1 tsp. whole cumin seeds

1 tsp. mustard seeds

1 tsp. kosher or rock salt*

1 pinch *hing* (asafoetida)

7–10 cups water

*Bragg Liquid Aminos can be added after cooking for flavor or to replace salt.

Wash beans and rice together until water runs clear. In a large pot on medium heat mix ghee, mustard seeds, turmeric, *hing,* ginger, cumin seeds, cumin powder, and coriander powder, and stir together for a few minutes. Add rice and beans and stir again. Add the water and salt and bring to a boil. Boil for 10 minutes. Turn heat to low, cover pot, and continue to cook until rice and beans become soft (about 30–40 minutes). Add the cilantro leaves just before serving.

NUTS AND SEEDS

Mainly harvested in the fall, nuts and seeds are loaded with minerals, fat, and protein, making them the perfect food for winter. They strengthen the nervous and reproductive systems and build muscle, bone, and blood. Nuts do not combine well with starchy vegetables such as potatoes or beans, but they do combine easily with dairy and in small amounts with fruits and grains. Like beans, nuts can be hard to digest and may be soaked overnight and their thin skin peeled if possible. Almonds, soaked and peeled, are one of the best sources of nonanimal protein. Nut milks made by pulverizing nuts in a blender with a little water render their nutrients more available for assimilation. Light-roasting nuts is good in winter, but they are best eaten raw in summer and spring. Dry-roasting is especially bad in winter. Nut butters are hard to digest and should be taken in small doses with spices to aid digestibility, and should not be eaten at night.

DAIRY

Humans are the only mammal that continues to drink the milk of another species, or to drink milk at all after infancy. Many cultures never drank milk, especially in Asia and Africa, and so they will be likely to have a more difficult time drinking it. Although some ethnic groups do not have the enzymes to digest milk, by far the biggest problem with dairy products among most ethnic groups in this country is the way Americans consume the two most common forms of dairy—as cold milk on cereal and in ice cream. Cheese and butter are also very common in the American diet, and we do put quite a bit of milk in our coffee and tea, but cold milk and ice cream create the most trouble.

In traditional cultures in such places as Switzerland, India, and other agriculture-based communities, milk is rarely used cold. The milk is taken from the cow to the table and drunk raw, unhomogenized, and warm. In the industrialized West, we begin by taking milk from cows that have been injected with growth hormones and antibiotics to enhance yield and fed a diet loaded with pesticides. We then pasteurize the milk to kill anything the antibiotics might have missed, and for our total convenience we homogenize it so the cream doesn't separate out. During homogenization, the milk is blasted through a tiny filter at extremely high pressure, destroying the natural enzymes in the milk that make it digestible. According to Annemarie Colbin, the founder of the Natural Gourmet Cooking School, the increased onset of hardening arteries in this century is directly linked to the homogenized process. (The term "homogenized" almost always has a negative connotation when applied to art, literature, or design, yet was presumed to be a good thing when associated with milk!)

In the United States, lactose intolerance rose with cholesterol levels and obesity in the 1950s and '60s, just as homogenization of milk was becoming widespread. Pasteurization, a heating process to kill bacteria, was introduced to prevent disease, and although it alters milk from its natural state, it does not seem to be as bad for the milk as homogenization. (Pasteurization does, however, kill up to half of the vitamin C in milk.) Many states allow the sale of unhomogenized and even unpasteurized or "raw" milk, but if you intend to buy milk this way you should get to know the farm and the hygiene used around the farm before purchasing milk for your family. Many health food stores carry either raw or unhomogenized milk. There is no state law that the milk has to be homogenized, and each state has different laws with regard to pasteurization. If you have difficulty finding nonhomogenized milk, try spicing it and taking it warm or hot. Traditional cultures still commonly drink warm milk before bed, usually spiced with ginger, cardamom, cinnamon, mustard seed, cayenne, cumin, or honey, all of which help to break down milk's mucus-producing properties.

Try not to drink milk cold in the morning, when the digestion is slowest. The best way to give your children a cold in the winter or spring is to feed them cold cow's milk on cereal or in milk shakes, especially in the spring. Milk does not combine well with other foods, can cause digestive problems, and is high in mucus-producing properties, which refrigeration dramatically increases. The spices in hot milk, however, help to push open blocked sinuses and have a demulcent or lubricating effect that combats the drying tendencies of winter. I don't use this recipe much on my children or patients, though, preferring herbs to accomplish the same thing without the risk of contributing to mucus production. The best time of year to enjoy milk is in the summer, when milk's cooling properties act as a natural antidote to the heat. But when you culture milk to make cheese, yogurt, or buttermilk, it goes from a cooling food to a heating food. The yogurt heats up the digestive fires—unlike milk, which would put out the same fires. That is why Indian restaurants often serve a yogurt drink called *lassi* with the meal. (See the Glossary of Foods, Appendix 1, for details on dairy products.)

In the end, the decision whether to use dairy products or not is up to you and should be based on how well your body digests these foods. In general, try to drink milk warm in winter, restrict whole milk or use only small amounts of nonfat milk in spring, and always try to drink it in unhomogenized form.

MEAT

The debate continues to rage over whether the human body was designed to eat meat or not. One argument holds that human physiology most closely resembles that of herbivores, animals that consume mainly vegetation, or frugivores, who live mainly on fruit. Our hands are ideal for plucking and peeling fruit, this argument goes, and our teeth seem most appropriate for breaking husks and grinding cellulose-laden vegetables. The 22-foot-long human intestines are ideal for digesting raw fruit and vegetables, but their length can allow flesh foods to decay and toxify before they are fully digested. Carnivores have teeth and claws designed for tearing the flesh of their prey, and short digestive tracts that do not allow meat sufficient time to rot and become toxic during digestion. And since animals do not cook their meat, it passes even more quickly through their systems. Vegetarians argue that our ancestors ate meat as a last recourse and only very recently in our evolution. According to the opposing argument, humans are omnivores, capable of digesting fruits, vegetables, grains, seafood, and meat. Our most distant ancestors who had the capacity to make tools and use fire have been eating meat perhaps for millions of years. Who is right?

I believe that if we look back far enough in human history, we will find that our earliest ancestors ate primarily the abundant raw fruit and wild vegetation they found in the tropical zones of Africa where human life probably began. As the land of their origins became overpopulated, our ancestors migrated farther north and south of the equatorial regions where fruit and vegetation still grew in profusion. By the close of the last Ice Age 10,000 years ago, what is now northern and central Europe had become a cold and forbidding place where animals such as the woolly mammoth provided migrating, nomadic tribes of hunter-gatherers the most abundant source of food. Hunting was at best an unreliable source of provisions, however. The discovery of agriculture somewhere between 7,000 and 10,000 years ago gave humans the option of shifting the balance away from meat. Grains such as corn, wheat, rice, barley, and oats, which could be stored through the winter in dried form and consumed until spring, allowed tribes to remain in one place and develop stable cultures.

Some nutritionists insist that 10,000 years is not long enough for the human digestive system to have adapted to eating grains, and that even these wonderful foods should be avoided or minimized. The reality is that just as grains serve a valuable nutritional function when consumed under the proper circumstances, meat can also find a place in a healthful diet. Until very recently in the United States, it was almost impossible to eat a decent meal in most restaurants without ordering meat, fish, or poultry in some form. On top of that, making vegetarian meals is labor intensive and time consuming. I will give my recommendations for those who wish to pursue a meat-free diet as we go along. For now, let me acknowledge that there have historically been times and places where eating meat was an absolute necessity to survive. Although Buddhism, with its precept not to harm any sentient being, has traditionally promoted vegetarianism, even the Dalai Lama has admitted that he suffers from low energy and anemia if he doesn't eat some meat. In his homeland of Tibet, Buddhist monks ate meat because little vegetation grows on the cold and barren plateaus that make up much of the country. And if you had lived in Vermont 100 years ago, in the winter you would either have eaten meat or died.

The argument against eating meat is also compelling, however. The one animal that has a digestive system most closely approximating our own is the gorilla. Like humans, these animals have an acid stomach, an alkaline intestine that is about 22 feet long, and even the same number of teeth; our digestive systems are alike in every way. Yet gorillas are vegetarians, living exclusively on a diet of vegetation and fruit, and are among the most powerful beasts on earth; the only predator that seriously threatens their survival is humanity.

Does that mean that we should also be vegetarians? To begin with, gorillas have to consume enormous amounts of food to maintain their energy and size, and their diet is clearly one that could be maintained only in the tropics, where edible vegetation is abundant and the gorilla population is small. Most of humanity no longer lives in areas where a constant supply of mangoes, bananas, leaves, and roots is available in abundance. Given our busy Western lifestyle, vegetarianism is much more of a challenge than it was for our ancestors, and will vary with location. It is easier to be a vegetarian if you live in Bermuda, Florida, or Southern California than, say, Vermont or Montana, where not much grows in the winter. Constitution also plays a part: Winter types who live in the north need more protein, especially animal protein, and do not do so well on a raw or "live" food diet. Even genetics can determine how well one will adapt to vegetarianism. Some nutritionists believe that blood type, derived ultimately from one's ancestry, may affect your need for meat. If your direct ancestors came from the Mediterranean region— Italy, Greece, North Africa—you may be predisposed to a diet of fish, fruits, salads, and grains (including the processed grains of pasta and couscous). Those who trace their blood lines back to Scandinavia, Northern Europe, or the plains of Argentina might be more genetically predisposed to a diet heavy in meat.

I contend that we have all evolved dramatically since our blood types were cast, however, and after millennia of migration and intermarriage, some of us who have a classic meat-eating O blood type may not need meat at all. I am an O blood type and seem to do perfectly fine without meat.

If you are considering becoming a vegetarian, I urge you to use the same principle I expound in this book regarding which diet to eat. If you follow my 3-Season Diet, soon you will crave exactly what you need and what is being harvested. When this begins to happen, you do not need a research paper to tell you that you are eating correctly. You will know it, just as the birds know to fly south. If you are slowly losing the desire for meat, then you should give yourself permission to eat less—not because a book told you that you should or shouldn't. I recommend eating less meat starting in the spring or summer, when we naturally need and desire less protein and less heavy food. Come winter, make sure that you eat more protein in the form of nuts, seeds, tofu, and other high-protein vegetarian food, so your body can store it for a long spring and summer without becoming protein deficient. This transition process should be gentle and slow, and only if you are sure you are doing it because your body wants it, not because your mind thinks it is more healthful or the morally right thing to do. If it is right for you, it will stick. And if you are a vegetarian, give yourself permission to eat meat if you so desire. There are no absolutes here; even gorillas will eat meat on occasion when provoked or hungry enough. Let your body dictate what you need.

I recently gave a lecture on the digestive system to my daughter's fourth-grade class. When the subject of vegetarianism came up, I made a few points about the health benefits of not eating meat, but added that this has to be a personal decision. Some kids, I have found, naturally refuse to eat meat because they don't like seeing blood, and they should be allowed to trust their instincts. When I mentioned that cattle are slaughtered in large numbers just so we can eat at McDonald's, a child raised his hand and said that you don't have to kill an animal to eat a hamburger. Like so many kids today he had either never thought about it or had blocked out the connection between the slaughterhouse and the Big Mac. I believe that if we personally had to kill an animal to eat meat, we would not eat as much of it as we do today.

A writer named Suzanne Winckler has described her decision with a friend to raise and slaughter their own chickens every few years. "Butchering chickens is no fun," she writes, "which is one reason I do it. It is the price I pay for being an omnivore and for eating other meat, like beef and pork, for which I have not yet determined a workable way to kill." She also needs to "dispense with the layers of anonymous people between me and my food," but in the process finds herself connecting to previous generations who hunted and killed their own food "both as a necessity and an ordinary event," as well as to the more savage life of our distant ancestors. In the end she declares, "I am too far gone in my rational Western head to appropriate the ritual of cultures for whom the bloody business of hunting was a matter of survival. But butchering chickens has permitted me to stand in the black night just outside the edge of their campfire, and from that prospect I have inherited the most important lesson of all in the task of killing meat: I have learned to say thank you and I'm sorry."

In the summer, when fruits and vegetables are abundant, our natural tendency is to eat less meat. Think of native peoples; when trees were full of fruit and the ground rich with vegetables in spring and summer, you would not find them hunting and eating as much meat as in winter, when meat was pretty much all there was. This makes much more sense in the natural scheme of things than our habit of eating large amounts of meat all year round. When the climate in most of North America is cold and dry in winter, however, meat acts as an antidote. During the cold winter season, many animals hibernate to survive; their metabolism slows down and they need less energy. The foods that nature provides during this time for those of us not hibernating—including nuts, grains, root veggies, and meats—are heavier, higher in protein and fat. (Remember that protein foods build the body up, which is why body builders live on protein powders and amino acids to build muscle bulk.) The body actively seeks to store fat, protein, minerals, and vitamins all winter long, and it's perfectly natural to gain 5 pounds or so in this season, only to burn it off in the spring. If we do not provide those nutrients in the winter our body will be unsatisfied and will crave inappropriate foods the rest of the year. Many vegetarians find themselves protein deficient in the winter because they fail to adjust their diets accordingly. If they are not careful about their diet, they can become addicted to sugar for their nutritional energy, instead of getting it from a well-balanced diet free of flesh foods. Vegetarians often complain of hypoglycemia and fluctuating energy levels, while they secretly binge on chocolates for energy. Their low energy does not result from meatless meals, however, but from an imbalance in their diet. If you are on any diet, whether vegetarian or high protein, please look at your cravings. Are you satisfied and not craving anything or are you constantly longing for foods that are "off the diet"? Proteins burn slowly and are heavy and calming. If you are a vegetarian, you *can* get adequate protein. It just takes some foresight and preparation, a willingness to learn how to cook tofu and beans, and a bit of extra time.

Failing to eat the foods that nature provides for each season can have other consequences for health as well. One October not long ago, I began to suffer excruciating neck pain from a car accident that had occurred 10 years before. As the pain grew progressively worse, I sought out a variety of complementary medical treatments. Chiropractic, neuromuscular and cranial-sacral therapy, rolfing, and massage all provided temporary relief, but the pain always returned. Then it dawned on me that the winter season had begun, yet I was still cruising along on my regular diet, having forgotten to increase my protein intake. That day I drank three protein shakes and woke up the next morning with absolutely no neck pain. I continued to eat plenty of protein and the pain never recurred. Could there actually have been a nutritional reason for my pain?

When the body is deficient in protein it is believed that one of the first places it looks within itself to satisfy its needs is the synovial fluid of the joints. When the body is forced to extract too much protein from this source, the fluid dries up and the blood supply to the joints is cut off. As a result the body begins to lay down a tougher kind of tissue that doesn't need blood—what we call scar tissue. This tougher scar tissue renders the joints stiff and painful. Increasing my protein intake allowed the high-protein synovial fluid that had been depleted from my neck to reestablish itself, and my pain disappeared.

If you are a vegetarian and you get winter aches and pains, you may want to check your protein levels. If you are having joint trouble but are against eating meat, than take a protein powder; sometimes the soy powders are hard to digest, so try a whey protein powder, which is light and relatively easy to digest.

HERBAL TIP

I F MUSCULAR ACHES are chronic because the body has been protein deficient for a prolonged time, you may need some heavy artillery to break down the scar tissue and reestablish the blood flow to the joints. An herb called boswella, a digestion-friendly anti-inflammatory that also breaks up scar tissue, has been shown in studies to relieve 85 percent of cases with chronic joint pain. Boswella doesn't only relieve inflammation but also increases blood supply to the joint capsule that is lost during periods of protein deficiency and scar tissue build-up. It comes in a tablet (boswellic acid) for internal consumption, and is readily available in any vitamin store. According to one study, it should be taken at 300 mg three times a day for six weeks to show significant pain relief. It also comes in a topical cream that works almost immediately; I recommend taking both.

NATURE'S ANTIDOTE

As Native American and ancient Asian cultures have long proposed, nature is neither static nor haphazard but moves in cycles that flow effortlessly and organically into one another. The ancient Vedas of India describe the universe as a continuous process of creation, destruction, and rebirth. In the ancient Chinese symbol for yin and yang, the white dot within a black swirl represents the seed of the white swirl that makes up the other half of the circle. Likewise, during each of the three seasonal harvests that make up the annual cycle, nature produces the seeds with which to heal the ills of that season and help prepare the body for the season that follows. I call these seeds nature's antidote. In the West we look on nature as a cruel force that must be subdued through technological wizardry, but the Native American and Eastern traditions see in nature the potential solutions to every imbalance.

THE SPRING ANTIDOTE DIET

Pam was going into her second year on my 3-Season Diet, making changes in her old eating habits gradually and gracefully. Rather than adhering to a rigid list of prescribed foods, she was allowing her own growing desire for the right foods to lead her along the way. Her long history of constipation was becoming regulated naturally, without laxatives or enemas. As a result Pam's energy level and her moods, marked by a tendency toward depression, had stabilized. Then one day in mid-March, she came to see me complaining of a loss of appetite. I asked her if she had been craving anything, and when she thought about it for a moment, her face lit up with recognition.

"Yes," she said, "I'm craving salads like crazy!"

I smiled appreciatively and said that was good. Checking for other symptoms, I determined that she had not been gaining weight and that her moods and energy levels were fine. Lack of appetite was her only complaint. I told her that, far from being a problem, it was perfectly natural for her appetite to trail off when it did. At the end of a long winter, the body has become increasingly dried out and has produced excessive mucus, a potential cause of colds. After having sought to counteract the dryness of winter by eating heavy, fatty foods rich in protein, it's now time for the cycle to revolve again. Spring is nature's new year, the time to make new resolutions to burn fat because the body is not getting it from anywhere else. Think of the birds: They set up house in the spring and prepare for the nestlings that will soon arrive. The chicks must grow to maturity in the four short months of summer and be strong enough to fly south in winter and begin the cycle again.

Turning up the heat, nature provides water and mud to help germinate seeds and prepare for the growing season. The only problem with all the moisture and mud is that it can become excessive if you continue eating heavy winter foods, especially if you have a spring constitution. If in winter we counteracted dryness with wet, sweet foods, in spring the problem is reversed, and nature provides an antidote to all the moisture in the form of cold vegetables and bitter and astringent foods like peas, leafy greens, and root vegetables that clean and detoxify the body. Before we had refrigerators, we ate roots like echinacea, dandelion, golden seal, burdock root, and Oregon grape. Today we think of those as medicines, but we can eat foods that have a similar taste: bitter, astringent, and pungent (spicy).

The moisture of spring that softened the ground and opened it up so that seeds can germinate and plants can grow in summer also softens and opens up the tissues of our bodies. This is the perfect time for detoxification and cleansing, which is why mystics and Native Americans traditionally go on spring fasts and why Lenten fasting is part of the Christian tradition. As a Catholic boy growing up in the Northeast, I was encouraged to "give up" candy or something I liked for Lent. This was presented as a way of doing something pleasing to God, and yet I believe that this tradition is derived from an ancient, seasonal-based practice of cleansing the body in spring (which is certainly pleasing to the Divine as well). Along with bitter, astringent, and pungent foods, we can use chlorophyll, the pigment that gives plants their green color, as a potent natural internal cleanser in either tablet or liquid form. Mix a tablespoonful in a glass of water every morning before eating—it's also an excellent deodorizer and breath freshener. Wheat grass juice, freshly pressed from the sprouting grasses of the wheat berry, is another useful supplement that you can get at many health food stores and natural juice bars.

Because seasons don't change overnight in nature, from winter snows one day to spring blooms the next, your diet doesn't need to change dramatically, either. You can introduce the changes I will outline below gradually and comfortably. Taper off your use of oils, red meat, nuts, and sweeteners in the spring; begin to introduce more of the bitter and astringent greens that you avoided in winter. In essence:

1. Favor foods that are light, dry, and warm. Minimize foods that are heavy, oily, and cold.
2. Favor foods that are spicy, bitter, and astringent. Minimize foods that are sweet, salty, and sour.

SOME SPECIFIC SPRING RECOMMENDATIONS

DAIRY. The best course is to avoid dairy products altogether in spring, substituting soy or rice milk. If you must have cow's milk, the low-fat or nonfat, nonhomogenized kind is best. Try to boil milk before you drink it to make it easier to digest, and take it warm. Do not take milk with a full meal or with sour or salty food. You might add one or two pinches of turmeric or powdered ginger to whole milk before drinking it to help reduce any spring-increasing qualities in the milk.

FRUITS. Although little fresh fruit is available naturally in the spring, you can eat cherries, blueberries, strawberries and other berries, and dried fruits such as raisins, prunes, and mulberries. Reduce heavy or sour fruits, such as oranges, bananas, pineapples, figs, dates, avocados, coconuts, and melons, as these fruits increase heaviness and the wet properties abundant in spring. Reduce everything, in brief, that you ate during the winter. Lighter fruits such as apples and pears are better for you.

SWEETENERS. Avoid sweeteners except uncooked honey. Reduce sugar products, as these increase spring qualities.

BEANS. All are fine; eat tofu in moderation.

NUTS. Reduce all nuts.

GRAINS. Emphasize barley, buckwheat, corn, rye, and millet. Do not take too much wheat or rice, as they increase spring qualities.

SPICES. All are fine, except for salt, which increases spring moisture.

VEGETABLES. Use bitter greens: radicchio, arugula, endive (a popular spring salad in French and Italian restaurants), dandelion greens, cabbage vegetables like broccoli and Brussels sprouts, green chilies, garlic, onions. Reduce tomatoes, cucumbers, sweet potatoes, and zucchini, which increase spring moisture.

Meat and Fish (FOR NONVEGETARIANS). White meat from chicken or turkey is fine. Freshwater fish or other light seafood (sole, flounder, rainbow trout) are all right in moderation. Reduce deep-sea fish such as tuna, halibut, swordfish, shark, and mahimahi, as well as shellfish, lobster, pork, and red meat. Eggs are acceptable in moderation but not fried, because of the excess oil and butter. Try eating them poached or hard-boiled instead.

OILS. Reduce use of oils. You have already stocked up on EFAs in winter, and what you need will come from grains and certain vegetables. Use mainly corn, safflower, sunflower, and soybean oil or a little ghee (clarified butter; see the Glossary of Foods, Appendix 1).

THE SUMMER ANTIDOTE DIET

The idea behind adjusting out diets to the seasons is to stay in the present moment, to understand what the seasons are doing to the body, and treat it accordingly with the foods that nature provides. Just as the earth holds on to more water from the rains of spring, the body holds on to more water during spring as well. These excess fluids, along with the natural increase of physical activity in spring, help to flush the body of seasonal toxins. Combined with a lower-fat harvest, this heightened activity also forces the body to increase its fat metabolism. By softening the tissues with its wet and rain, spring has given you access to them, and so during the spring, fat metabolism goes into high gear. Summer is a time of high energy, demanding the energy-producing properties of fruit, veggies, and other carbs. If you have eaten properly during spring, fat will continue to be a baseline energy source in the summer that will keep you on an even keel as you eat more fruits and carbs in general. If you hadn't forced the body into fat metabolism in the springtime, the body would be deconditioned to burn its own fat stores for energy, and would start to crave emergency fuel.

With a high-carb, high-sugar harvest naturally available in summer, if you have not reset the blood sugar in the spring by activating fat metabolism, then you will be more susceptible to the ups and downs in blood sugar. To avoid low blood sugar (hypoglycemia) and energy problems (fatigue and depression), you must understand how nature designed the prevention and cure for them. In the same way that winter brings cool relief from the heat of summer, and spring provides respite from a cold, dry winter by giving us moisture, summer produces the heat we need to dry up the excessive moisture and mucus of spring. And so in summer:

1. Favor foods that are cool and liquid. Minimize foods that are hot.
2. Favor foods that are sweet, bitter, or astringent. Minimize foods that create heat (spicy, salty, or sour).

SOME SPECIFIC SUMMER RECOMMENDATIONS

DAIRY. Milk, butter, and ghee are good. Reduce yogurt, salty cheese, sour cream, and cultured buttermilk (their sour tastes aggravate summer qualities). Nonhomogenized milk is best.

SWEETENERS. All unrefined sweeteners are good except honey and molasses.

OILS. Olive, soy, sunflower, and coconut oils are best. Reduce sesame, almond, and corn oils, all of which increase summer qualities.

GRAINS. Wheat, white rice, barley, and oats are good. Reduce corn, rye, millet, and brown rice.

FRUITS. Favor sweet fruits, such as grapes, cherries, melons, avocados, coconuts, pomegranates, mangos, and sweet, fully ripened oranges, pineapples, and plums. Reduce sour fruits, such as grapefruit, unripe olives, papayas, and unripe pineapples and plums.

VEGETABLES. Favor asparagus, cucumbers, potatoes, green leafy vegetables, pumpkins, broccoli, cauliflower, celery, okra, lettuce, beans, green beans, zucchini. Reduce hot peppers, unripe tomatoes, carrots, beets, onions, garlic, radishes, and spinach.

SPICES. Coriander, mint, cardamom, and fennel are all right. But the following spices strongly increase heat and should be taken only in small amounts: ginger, cumin, black pepper, fenugreek, clove, celery seed, salt, and mustard seed. Chili peppers and cayenne should be avoided.

Meat and Fish (FOR NONVEGETARIANS). Since meat and heavier flesh foods produce heat, emphasize lighter flesh foods. Chicken, pheasant, and turkey are preferable to beef, lamb, and other red meat. Eat white-flesh, freshwater fish like trout or sole rather than heavier, deep-sea fish or shellfish, as the sea salt will heat the body. Egg yolks increase heat and should be eaten in moderation. Don't bother separating egg whites from yolks, though. Despite what many nutritionists say about egg yolks being a source of cholesterol, the yolk also contains lecithin, which helps keep cholesterol liquid in the bloodstream and ultimately reduces cholesterol levels. And as with milk, the egg is a whole food that is better consumed whole or avoided altogether. Once you start taking nature apart, you generally run into trouble. The real cause of cholesterol, as we have seen, is stress and the sedentary life that allows our lymph to stagnate. Free radicals in the lymphatic system oxidate the fats, which lodge in the arterial walls and create life-threatening plaque.

THE WINTER ANTIDOTE DIET

In winter, the cold and wind dry out the land. Our bodies become dried out, too, a sensation we can feel in our throats and sinuses. Often the first indication that a change has happened or that a cold is coming on is a scratchy throat or dried mucus in the sinuses. As a defense against the irritation caused in the membranes by allergens and pollutants, the body produces mucus. Unfortunately, this mucus becomes an ideal place for bacteria to accumulate and help cold and flu germs breed. To counteract the drying effects of winter, then, we draw on nature's high-protein, high-fat antidote in the form of warm, heavy, oily foods that will replenish our depleted reserves of moisture. This means heavy foods like bananas, avocados, beets, winter squash, nuts, meat, deep-sea fish, and more oils.

We also seek out foods that taste sweet, sour, and salty. Why these tastes? In each case, nature is providing something that the body needs to pacify the change of season. We've all seen how rock salt melts the ice on the frozen sidewalks and roadways of winter; salt heats up the body as well, so we increase our intake of salty foods and of salt itself. Because it heats the body, salt acts as a carrier to bring minerals and nutrients deep into the body's tissues. Most spices work well in the winter as they, too, typically have a heating quality that combats the cold. Sweet foods such as yams and sweet potatoes also open up and nourish the tissues, which helps to counteract the dryness and lightness in winter. These foods also tend to calm and pacify the body, especially when those winter winds rattle your bones. Foods that are sour in taste tend to heat the body and stimulate the digestion. Did you ever wonder why delis give you a slice of sour pickle with your pastrami sandwich? In the East people traditionally take pickled lemon and ginger before a meal to stimulate the fire in the digestive system. Sour foods such as oranges and grapefruits also contain plenty of water to counteract winter's dryness—and Florida happens to produce its most luscious citrus fruits just when we need them most.

In the world of naturopathic medicine, dairy products are forbidden on the principle that lactase, the enzyme that digests milk, is not produced in humans after infancy. Yet in the Ayurvedic system of nutrition which is based on thousands of years of natural wisdom about food, dairy products are promoted as a good source of nutrition. As I've already stated, I believe that the problem is not in milk but in the process of homogenization, which renders the fat in milk indigestible, and in the way we keep milk refrigerated. In European countries where milk is still consumed the traditional way, lactose intolerance is rare. During the spring, which is a naturally congestive time of year, milk should be avoided because it is congestive, more so if it is drunk cold and heavily processed. In winter I would also avoid milk, particularly for kids. A small amount can be taken if heated up with some ginger or cardamom, which make it soothing to the nervous system, especially before bedtime (another folk remedy that actually works). For many people, whole milk is probably more nutritious than low-fat or no-fat milk. Certain ethnic groups, such as Chinese and Africans, do not have the enzymes to digest milk and should avoid.

Especially in the northern tier of the United States, people associate apples and pears with fall, because that's when they appear in abundance in roadside farm stands and markets in the countryside. At the same time that apples and pears are being harvested in that part of the country, leaves on trees are turning bright red and then yellow. As heat rises through the trees during months of a process known as "thermal accumulation," it manifests in fiery color. But at the same time, the ripe produce of apple and peach and pear orchards falls to the ground and provides the antidote we need in the form of cooling fruit. If we go into the winter without having first cooled off, the combination of accumulated summer heat and the dryness of winter can be devastating to our health. These end-of-summer fruits are loaded with fiber, which helps to clean the intestinal tract and drive all the accumulated heat of the past four months out of the body through the organs of elimination, not allowing it to rise into our heads, drying us out and triggering mucus production and a susceptibility to colds and flu. Fresh apple juice especially acts as a mild natural laxative.

So as you ease into winter, start by eating copious amounts of seasonal fruit in the fall, then begin to eat more protein and fat, more hearty soups, grains, nuts, and meat if so inclined. In general:

1. Favor foods that are warm, heavy, and oily. Minimize foods that are cold, dry, and light.
2. Favor foods that are sweet, sour, and salty. Minimize foods that are spicy, bitter, and astringent, as these foods are light and cold and will increase these qualities in us.
3. Eat larger quantities of food, but not more than you can digest easily. More food provides more heat for the body when the weather is cold.

SOME SPECIFIC WINTER RECOMMENDATIONS

DAIRY. Children should avoid milk, and adults should use it in small amounts—and only those who are strong winter body types (see chapter

7) and tend to dry out in winter. Try to boil or heat milk before you drink it. Don't drink milk with a full meal. Nonhomogenized is preferred. To reduce its congestive properties, add ginger, turmeric, cardamom, black pepper, and honey or raw sugar to taste if needed. Eat cheese in moderation and only at the midday meal, as with all dairy products in winter, with the exception of a small cup of spiced hot milk before bed.

SWEETENERS. All natural sweeteners are good (in moderation).

OILS. All oils by their very nature reduce winter dryness and lightness.

GRAINS. Most grains, harvested in fall to be eaten in winter, are warming and sweet and are fine, although some are heavier and more warming than others. Rice, especially brown rice, and wheat are very good. Eat less barley, millet, corn, buckwheat, rye, and dry oats. Wheat has gluten, which in excess can create digestive problems, so balance your intake. If winter is the time to load up on protein, you may wonder why I'm recommending an increase in grains, which are essentially carbohydrates. The reason is that grains contain more essential fatty acids than high-carb foods like vegetables, and some grains, such as amaranth, are as much as 25 percent protein.

FRUITS. Favor sweet, sour, or heavy fruits, such as oranges, bananas, avocados, grapes, grapefruit, cherries, peaches, plums, pineapples, mangos, and papayas. Apples and pears are great at the end of summer as we make the transition into winter. Think of the apples on a tree. They fall and are good for a short time; if we did not refrigerate them, they would rot in three weeks. After that time, as we go into winter eat cooked apples or sour varieties, which will have a more heating, antiwinter effect. I like apples with yogurt and honey in the morning, which is a warming combination. The apple is well balanced for winter when surrounded by heating foods. Reduce dry or light fruits such as pomegranates and cranberries, and dried fruits.

VEGETABLES. Beets, carrots, winter squash, acorn squash, tomatoes, okra, onions, artichoke hearts, and sweet potatoes are good, but should be cooked, not raw. The following vegetables are acceptable in moderate quantities if they're well cooked, rather than steamed, especially with ghee or oil and winter-reducing spices: peas, broccoli, cauliflower, celery, zucchini, and potatoes. It's better to avoid sprouts and cabbage and the bitter leafy greens, which are mainly spring and summer foods; if you must have them, be sure to cook them well.

SPICES. Cardamom, cumin, ginger, cinnamon, fennel, salt, cloves, mustard seed, and small quantities of black pepper are acceptable.

NUTS. All nuts are good.

BEANS. Reduce all beans, except for tofu and mung dal (a soup made from split dried mung beans). Winter is a time of high winds, so we don't want to eat foods that create *more* wind. Beans have a tendency to make us gassy and should be avoided. Besides, most beans absorb large amounts of water, and the last thing you need in winter is food that dehydrates you! If you want to eat beans, however (and I admit that hearty black bean soup can feel good on a cold day), make sure to soak them overnight, or cook them with three or four times the amount of water you normally would so that the beans absorb water that way, rather than taking it from you. This soaking will reduce their drying, wind-producing qualities. They can be spiced with antigas agents such as hing, fennel, ginger, and cardamom.

MEAT AND FISH (FOR NONVEGETARIANS). Chicken, turkey, and seafood, including heavier shellfish and lobster, are all right. If you are going to eat red meat, this is the time of year to indulge that desire, when the body needs heat. Remember, winter is the time to store fats, proteins, and minerals so that you will have abundant energy for the change into spring. In fact, after all the protein-rich, heavy, oily foods of winter, you will naturally crave a lighter diet rich in raw, leafy green vegetables. You won't have to "starve" yourself or struggle to eat greens as the weather turns warmer.

CHAPTER 5

Recipe Suggestions and Food Lists for the Seasons

T O GET YOU INTO the rhythm of eating what's appropriate for each season, I've prepared five sample menus each for spring, summer, and winter. These are just suggestions to give you an idea of what some typical days will look like on my program. As I've said before, I don't expect anyone to follow these outlines rigidly. If on any given day you simply don't have time or opportunity to eat your main meal at midday, then you can switch the supper and lunch menus. And since I know that not everyone is not a vegetarian, I've supplied nonvegetarian alternatives for the big meal of the day, so you can take your pick. But even if you're not vegetarian, I'd recommend trying one of the veggie dishes occasionally, just to see how you like them. You can also try to eat more of the vegetarian meals in the spring and summer and the meat meals in the winter to see if this suits your natural craving. These meals are easy to prepare and many are staples in our house. You may mix and match meals within a season or choose from the 3-Season Grocery List at the end of this chapter and design your own meal plan. Remember that in the 3-Season Diet, there are no bad foods (except fast food or overly processed foods). If you don't see a certain food that you especially love, just wait a few months and it will probably appear on the next season's grocery list. In time, you will be craving the foods on the list for the season you are in, and eating the appropriate food will once again become automatic.

Since it is not always possible to eat a large meal at midday, just use what I call the 51 Percent Principle: **As long as you eat this way the majority of the time, you will benefit from this program.** (I describe the 51 Percent Principle in much greater detail in Ch apter 9.) Soon it will become your preference to eat with the seasons and with the natural rhythms of your body. It is also human nature occasionally to eat pizza and ice cream or some such food combo that we know is not great for us. It's more important to do the right thing most of the time than to agonize over an occasional lapse, especially if you find yourself out with family and friends. To help offset the downside of such meals, try to break the rules around the midday meal rather than at night, for reasons I will make plain in the next chapter. If you do break the rules at night or even during the day, you can help out your digestive system with some of the tips I will mention later.

Following the sample menus below, I've included a master list of all the foods that are appropriate to eat in each of the seasons at the end of this chapter. You can tape this and the grocery list in Appendix 3 to your refrigerator for ready reference to begin with. After a short time they will become second nature, and you will find yourself craving the right foods at the right time of year.

The following menus are designed to be a way of life rather than a six-month diet to lose thirty pounds. By eating according to these menus you will lose weight. It will come off gracefully and permanently. If you want to accelerate the weight loss using this program, see Part II, The Weight Balancing Program, where the 3-season diet is combined with techniques to reset the body's ability to burn fat as the primary fuel supply.

SPRING
Lower-Fat, Lower-Calorie Diet

(March–June)

DAY ONE

BREAKFAST
GRAPEFRUIT WITH HONEY
RYE TOAST WITH APPLE BUTTER
FRESH CARROT, BEET, AND APPLE JUICE

LUNCH
BARLEY VEGETABLE SOUP (MADE WITH BARLEY, CARROTS,
GREEN BEANS, CELERY, DANDELIONS, MUSHROOMS, AND
ONIONS MIXED IN BLENDER) WITH RYE TOAST
STEAMED KALE (WITH BALSAMIC VINEGAR, CANOLA OIL, BLACK
PEPPER, AND GARLIC)
VEG: BAKED BEANS (WITH BASMATI RICE AND ASPARAGUS)
NONVEG: GRILLED CHICKEN BREAST (SKINLESS AND
BONELESS, MARINATED IN GINGER-TAMARI SAUCE AND
GRILLED)

SUPPER
SPLIT PEA SOUP (MADE WITH BARLEY AND CARROTS, CELERY,
ONIONS, AND GARLIC)
TOASTED RYE BREAD

DAY TWO

BREAKFAST

Low-Fat Yogurt (mixed with honey, raisins, papaya,
apples, and pumpkin seeds)
Freshly Juiced Apple-Celery Juice

LUNCH

Mixed Green Salad (made with papaya slices, poppy
seed dressing, canola, or sunflower oil)
Sautéed Mixed Greens (made with dandelions, spinach,
and mustard greens sautéed in safflower oil with
garlic and onions)
VEG: Garbanzo Bean Casserole (made with cornmeal,
carrots, onions, fresh corn, tomato sauce, cayenne,
coriander, and sage)
NONVEG: Broiled Fillet of Salmon (rubbed with a
mixture of ginger, cumin, cayenne, paprika, cinnamon,
anise, and turmeric and broiled)

SUPPER

Cream of Spinach Soup (made with Rice Dream, ginger,
paprika, black pepper, and cooked spinach, blended
and cooled)
Corn Bread

DAY THREE

BREAKFAST
GRITS (CORNMEAL CEREAL WITH HONEY)
RAW APPLES AND PEARS (SLICED WITH HONEY AND
CINNAMON)
GRAPEFRUIT WITH HONEY
HERBAL TEA
FRESH CARROT JUICE

LUNCH
SPINACH SALAD (MADE WITH SLICED MUSHROOMS AND
VINAIGRETTE DRESSING)
STEAMED ARTICHOKE (WITH OREGANO, BASIL, BAY LEAF, AND
MARJORAM)
MIXED GREEN VEGETABLES (STEAMED GREEN BEANS,
CABBAGE, AND BROCCOLI WITH MARJORAM AND PUREED
TURNIPS AND CARROTS)
VEG: INDIAN-STYLE RICE AND BEANS (LONG-GRAIN BROWN
RICE AND SPLIT MUNG BEANS WITH TURMERIC, GINGER, AND
BLACK PEPPER)
NONVEG: FILLET OF SOLE OR FLOUNDER (BRAISED IN LIGHT
CHICKEN BROTH, FINELY SLICED LEEKS, AND MINCED
SHALLOTS)

SUPPER
GARBANZO SOUP (MADE WITH PUREED GARBANZO BEANS AND
CHOPPED ASPARAGUS, HING, CUMIN, CAYENNE, GARLIC, AND
CORIANDER, SPRINKLED WITH FRESH CILANTRO AND LEMON)
CHOPPED ASPARAGUS (TOPPED WITH FRESH PARSLEY)
BARLEY OR RYE TOAST OR FLAT BREAD

DAY FOUR

BREAKFAST

HOT BARLEY CEREAL (MIXED WITH HONEY AND CHOICE OF
DRIED FRUITS, APPLES, OR RAISINS)
FRESH* GRAPEFRUIT JUICE

LUNCH

CARROT SOUP
SPINACH SALAD (MADE WITH ROASTED PINE NUTS AND
CURRANTS OR RAISINS, WITH RASPBERRY VINAIGRETTE
DRESSING)
VEG: PESTO PASTA (WITH STEAMED SNOW PEAS ON THE SIDE)
NONVEG: BAKED TURKEY (WITH MASHED POTATOES AND
SNOW PEAS)

SUPPER

CORN CHOWDER (MADE WITH CELERY, ONIONS, AND
POTATOES)
CORN BREAD AND HONEY

---

*Whenever possible.

DAY FIVE

BREAKFAST

Fresh Fruit Salad (papaya, blueberries, strawberries, raspberries, blackberries, and apples)
Rye Toast or Corn Bread with Honey
Hot Water with Lemon and Honey

LUNCH

Steamed Broccoli or Green Beans (with baked potato and sour cream)
VEG: Stuffed Bell Peppers (stuffed with quinoa cooked in vegetable or chicken broth, shredded carrots, and mushrooms with your choice of spring spices)
Alfalfa and Mung Bean Sprout Salad (with honey-lemon dressing)
NONVEG: Fillet of Rainbow Trout (baked in lemon juice, white wine, salt, freshly ground black pepper, and spices from spring spice list)

SUPPER

Vegetarian Chili with Corn Bread

Spring Teas
Cinnamon, Ginger, Black Tea, Green Tea, Raspberry Leaf

Spring Snacks
Corn Chips, Dried Fruits, Berries, Sprouts, Carrots, Pumpkin Seeds, Apple, Grapefruit

Spring Spices
See spice list, pages 116–117

SUMMER
High-Carb Diet

July–October

DAY ONE

BREAKFAST
FRESH FRUIT SALAD (GRAPES, MANGOES, BLUEBERRIES,
APPLES, PAPAYA, TOPPED WITH SHREDDED COCONUT AND
CHOPPED MACADAMIA NUTS)
WHOLE-GRAIN TOAST (WITH BUTTER OR APPLE BUTTER)
FRESH-PRESSED APPLE JUICE
HERB TEA

LUNCH
CUCUMBER-MINT GAZPACHO
BASMATI RICE (WITH TOASTED PUMPKIN SEEDS AND
SHREDDED COCONUT)
ROASTED ASPARAGUS (COATED WITH OLIVE OIL, LEMON, AND
HING)
GARBANZO BEANS (MADE WITH TOMATOES, TURMERIC, RAW
SUGAR, GHEE, AND CILANTRO)
SAUTÉED BROCCOLI (WITH GHEE, SALT, HING)
VEG: PAN-ROASTED TOFU (CUBED AND BROWNED WITH OLIVE
OIL, RAW SUGAR, AND BRAGG LIQUID AMINOS)
NONVEG: BROILED FRESHWATER SALMON (WITH ORANGE MINT
MARMALADE)

SUPPER
STEAMED ARTICHOKE (COOKED WITH CORIANDER AND FENNEL
SEEDS, WITH LEMON BUTTER DIP)
PEA SOUP (MADE WITH FRESH PEAS,* RICE DREAM,
PAPRIKA, AND BUTTER)

---

*If fresh are not available, use frozen, but avoid canned peas.

DAY TWO

BREAKFAST

CREAM OF WHITE RICE CEREAL (MADE WITH HOT MILK, OR
RICE OR SOY MILK, AND SLICED BANANA, SWEETENED WITH
CHOPPED DATES, SUCANAT, OR HONEY)
FRESH-SQUEEZED ORANGE JUICE

LUNCH

MIXED GREEN SALAD (LETTUCE, ALFALFA SPROUTS,
CUCUMBERS, AND WATERCRESS, WITH RASPBERRY JUICE AND
OLIVE OIL)
CHILLED FENNEL-AND-APPLE GAZPACHO
VEG: STUFFED BELL PEPPER (WITH BASMATI RICE, GHEE,
CELERY, KIDNEY BEANS, AND CHOPPED CILANTRO)
NONVEG: COBB SALAD (ADD SLICED GRILLED CHICKEN AND
SMALL AMOUNT OF CRUMBLED BLUE CHEESE TO A MIXED
GREEN SALAD)

SUPPER

CREAM OF POTATO AND RED PEPPER SOUP (MADE WITH RICE
DREAM)
MIXED GREEN SALAD

DAY THREE

BREAKFAST

3-Fruit Juice (fresh juice of pineapple, orange, and guava in equal parts)

Rye Toast with Fruit Spread

Oatmeal

LUNCH

Melon-and-Orange-Juice gazpacho (topped with raspberries)

Cucumber Salad

VEG: Lemon-Broiled Tofu (with broiled red and yellow peppers and zucchini)

NONVEG: Fillet of Rainbow Trout (braised in chicken broth and sliced leeks)

Basmati Rice

Steamed Chopped Zucchini, Asparagus, and Broccoli

SUPPER

Fresh Fruit Salad

Cream of Mushroom Soup (sauté mushrooms in butter, add black pepper and Rice Dream, and blend)

DAY FOUR

BREAKFAST

CANTALOUPE AND HONEYDEW MELON (WITH A SQUEEZE OF
ORANGE)
SOURDOUGH WHEAT TOAST
HERB TEA

LUNCH

VEG: VEGGIE SHISH KEBOB (CHERRY TOMATOES, PINEAPPLE,
AND TOFU ON SKEWERS, GRILLED, WITH BASMATI RICE)
NONVEG: SHISH KEBOB (CHERRY TOMATOES, PINEAPPLE, AND
SHRIMP ON SKEWERS, WITH BASMATI RICE)
ZUCCHINI (WITH A TOUCH OF GHEE)
STEAMED SNOW PEAS (WITH TOUCH OF GHEE)
WATERMELON

SUPPER

SPLIT PEA SOUP
PIECE OF SOURDOUGH OR ITALIAN BREAD

DAY FIVE

BREAKFAST

GRANOLA (WITH ORANGE JUICE OR MILK, BANANA, AND
BERRIES) OR GRANOLA (WITH PEACHES AND MILK, OR RICE OR
SOY MILK)
HERB TEA

LUNCH

MINESTRONE SOUP
VEG: GARDEN BURGER (WITH TOMATO, LETTUCE, CUCUMBER,
AND BELL PEPPER)
NONVEG: TURKEY BURGER (WITH TOMATO, LETTUCE,
CUCUMBER, AND BELL PEPPER)
STEAMED BROCCOLI
SEASONAL FRUIT SALAD

SUPPER

COTTAGE CHEESE AND PEACHES
HERB TEA

Summer Teas

CHAMOMILE, PEPPERMINT, CORIANDER, GINGER, SPEARMINT,
CINNAMON, CARDAMOM, LICORICE, HIBISCUS,
STRAWBERRY LEAF

Summer Snacks

WATERMELON, RIPE FRUIT IN SEASON, ICE CREAM IN
MODERATION IN THE MIDDLE OF THE DAY AFTER LUNCH,
PEACHES, CELERY, COCONUT, GRAPES, APPLE,
MACADAMIA NUTS

Summer Spices

SEE SPICE LIST, PAGES 116–117

WINTER
Higher-Protein, Higher-Fat Diet

November–February

DAY ONE

BREAKFAST

YOGURT, PAPAYA AND/OR MANGO (WITH PURE MAPLE SYRUP
OR CHOPPED DATES WITH SLICED ALMONDS, WALNUTS, AND
PECANS)
TOAST (WITH APPLE BUTTER OR SMALL AMOUNT OF DAIRY
BUTTER)
HOT HERB TEA

LUNCH

AVOCADO-TOMATO SALAD (WITH ARTICHOKE HEARTS, FRESH
BASIL, FRESH MOZZARELLA, OLIVE OIL, AND VINEGAR)
ORANGE AND BEET SOUP (HEAT 3 TABLESPOONS OLIVE OIL IN
LARGE SAUCEPAN AND SAUTÉ 2 CELERY STALKS, 2 LARGE
CARROTS, 2 LARGE POTATOES, AND 3 MEDIUM BEETS FOR A
FEW MINUTES. ADD TEASPOON SALT AND CUP ORANGE JUICE
AND ENOUGH WATER TO COVER VEGETABLES. COOK UNTIL
VEGETABLES ARE TENDER. ADD FRESH GROUND BLACK PEPPER
AND SEA SALT TO TASTE.)
VEG: SPLIT YELLOW MUNG BEAN SOUP (WITH TOMATOES,
TURMERIC, CUMIN, GINGER, HING, CORIANDER, SALT, BLACK
PEPPER, OR CAYENNE)
NONVEG: BARBECUED OR BROILED HALIBUT (WITH LEMON)
BROWN OR BASMATI RICE (WITH COCONUT AND CASHEWS,
MUSTARD SEEDS, TURMERIC, CINNAMON, CLOVE, CORIANDER,
AND CUMIN)
STEAMED OKRA, BEETS, OR CARROTS, OR WELL-COOKED
BROCCOLI (WITH SLICED ALMONDS)
COOKIE

SUPPER

ACORN OR WINTER SQUASH SOUP (WITH COCONUT MILK, ONION, AND GARLIC)

TOASTED NONYEASTED FLAT BREAD (WITH BUTTER OR NUT BUTTER—*NOT* PEANUT BUTTER)

(NONYEASTED BREADS ARE EASIER TO DIGEST IN THE EVENING.)

DAY TWO

BREAKFAST

TOFU BURRITO (A BIG FLOUR OR CORN TORTILLA WITH MASHED
HARD TOFU, TOMATO, TURMERIC, SALT, GINGER, CUMIN,
CAYENNE, AND HING—OR BUY A READY-MIX TOFU SCRAMBLER)
HERB TEA (WITH NATURAL SWEETENER)
FRESH BEET AND CARROT JUICE

LUNCH

SWEET-POTATO AND COCONUT-MILK SOUP, OR CARROT-AND-
SWEET POTATO SOUP
VEG: BARBECUED OR GRILLED TOFU WITH BARBECUE SAUCE
(MADE WITH PINEAPPLE JUICE, TOMATO SAUCE, TABASCO, AND
RAW SUGAR)
NONVEG: BARBECUED OR PAN-SEARED TUNA (WITH GROUND
CORIANDER, FENNEL SEED, AND WHITE PEPPER CRUST)
MASHED POTATOES OR SWEET POTATOES, AND GINGERED
CARROTS

SUPPER

CARROT SOUP (MADE WITH ONION, POTATO, TOMATOES, AND
CURRY)
FLAT BREAD

DAY THREE

BREAKFAST

HOT WHOLE-GRAIN CEREAL (WHOLE WHEAT, RICE, OATS, OR MULTIGRAIN, WITH HONEY AND A SMALL AMOUNT OF HOT MILK OR RICE OR SOY MILK) (GRAINS CAN VARY, SINCE IN THE WINTER HOT CEREAL CAN BECOME A HABIT.)
ORANGE JUICE AND/OR TEA

LUNCH

POTATO AND CHEESE SOUP
VEG: ENCHILADAS (MADE WITH BROWN RICE, CHEESE, SOUR CREAM, BLACK OLIVES, TOMATOES, CAYENNE, CUMIN, HING, ONION, GARLIC, WITH AVOCADO AND MELTED SOY OR DAIRY CHEESE)
NONVEG: QUICHE LORRAINE (TOPPED WITH SOUR CREAM) OR CRAB QUICHE
SMALL SERVING OF SWEET OF YOUR CHOICE (PREFERABLY WITH NO REFINED SUGAR OR ARTIFICIAL SWEETENERS)

SUPPER

BORSCHT (SOUP MADE WITH BEETS, CABBAGE, AND SOUR CREAM)
WHOLE-GRAIN TOAST

DAY FOUR

BREAKFAST

EGGS ANY STYLE (WITH WHOLE-WHEAT, SOURDOUGH, OR
NONYEASTED TOAST WITH BUTTER)
ORANGE JUICE
HERB TEA

LUNCH

SMALL GREEN SALAD (WITH LEMON, SALT, HONEY, AND
GINGER DRESSING)
VEG: FETTUCCINE ALFREDO
NONVEG: SPAGHETTI CARBONARA (SAUTÉ WELL-COOKED
CARROTS AND BROCCOLI WITH ALMONDS IN OLIVE OIL OR
GHEE)

SUPPER

MUNG BEAN SOUP (MADE WITH CARROTS, POTATOES,
TOMATOES, ONIONS, AND CURRY)
ONE WHOLE-WHEAT CHAPATI

DAY FIVE

BREAKFAST
WHOLE-GRAIN WAFFLES (WITH PURE MAPLE SYRUP)
FRUIT MÉLANGE (DATES, BANANAS, MANGOES, PAPAYAS, AND GRAPES)
FRESH CARROT, BEET, AND APPLE JUICE
HERB TEA WITH HONEY

LUNCH
FRENCH ONION SOUP
VEG: FIVE-GRAIN TEMPEH (SLICE INTO 1-INCH CUBES, BROWN IN OIL AND BRAGG LIQUID AMINOS, ADD SOUR CREAM, AND TOSS FOR 1 MINUTE)
NONVEG: SHRIMP SCAMPI (WITH GRATED SWEET POTATO AND POWDERED GINGER AND GHEE, SAUTÉED UNTIL TENDER)
BROWN RICE WITH NUTS

SUPPER
VEG: GINGER-CARROT SOUP
NONVEG: CHICKEN NOODLE SOUP
AVOCADO SALAD (WITH RICE WINE VINEGAR AND SALT)

Winter Teas
FENNEL, LICORICE, CARDAMOM, LEMON

Winter Snacks
NUTS, SMALL PORTION OF CHEESES, CARROTS OR WINTER FRUITS: GRAPES, MANGOES, BANANAS, PEARS, DATES

Winter Spices
SEE SPICE LIST, PAGES 116–117

3-Season Grocery List

GENERAL GUIDELINES

- In summer, eat off the summer list.
- In winter, eat off the winter list.
- In spring, eat off the spring list.
- Think in terms of increasing good foods in season rather than avoiding foods.
- Remember, there are no bad foods—if your favorite food does not appear in one season, wait a couple of months and it will show up on the next season's list.
- In spring, eat a low-fat diet by taking more salads, veggies, leafy greens, beans, sprouts, and berries.
- In summer, eat more fruits and veggies, as they are almost pure carbohydrates.
- In winter, eat more nuts, grains, soups, and meats to ensure the storage of protein and fats for the winter.
- Read chapter 7 to tailor the 3-Season Diet to your body type and geographic location.
- See the Glossary of Foods (Appendix 1) for details on common food.

KEY

1. Best   Best season for this food
2. Good   Second-best season for this food
3. Reduce   Eat small amounts, if any
4. Avoid   Try to eliminate this food

	SPRING	SUMMER	WINTER
Fruits			
Apples	Good	Best	Good, cooked
Apricots	Reduce, dried okay	Best	Good
Bananas	Reduce	Good	Best
Blueberries	Good	Best	Good

	SPRING	SUMMER	WINTER
Fruits			
Cantaloupe	Reduce	Best	Good w/lemon
Cherries	Reduce	Best, ripe	Good
Coconuts	Reduce	Best, green or ripe	Good, ripe
Cranberries	Reduce	Best	Good
Dates	Reduce	Good	Best
Dry Fruits	Best	Good	Reduce
Figs	Avoid	Good	Best
Grapefruit	Good	Reduce	Best
Grapes	Reduce, except raisins	Best	Best
Guava	Avoid	Best	Good
Lemons	Good	Reduce	Best
Limes	Good	Reduce	Best
Mangoes	Reduce	Best	Best
Melons	Reduce	Best	Reduce
Nectarines	Reduce	Good	Good
Oranges	Reduce	Good, sweet	Best
Papayas	Good	Good, sm. amts.	Best
Peaches	Reduce	Good, tree ripe	Good
Pears	Good	Best	Good, ripe
Persimmons	Reduce	Best	Best
Pineapples	Reduce	Best, sweet	Good
Plums	Reduce	Best, ripe	Good
Pomegranates	Good	Best	Reduce
Raspberries	Good	Best	Reduce
Strawberries	Good	Best	Good
Tangerines	Reduce	Good, sweet	Best
Vegetables			
Alfalfa Sprouts	Best	Good	Reduce
Artichokes	Good	Best	Good, hearts
Asparagus	Best	Best	Reduce
Avocados	Reduce	Good	Best
Bean Sprouts	Best	Good	Avoid

	SPRING	SUMMER	WINTER
Vegetables			
Beets	Good	Avoid, greens okay	Best
Bell Peppers	Best	Best	Reduce unless cooked
Bitter Melon	Good	Best	Reduce
Broccoli	Good	Best	Reduce unless cooked
Brussels Sprouts	Best	Avoid	Best
Cabbage	Best	Best	Avoid
Carrots	Best	Reduce	Best
Cauliflower	Best	Best	Avoid
Celery	Best	Best	Reduce unless cooked
Chicory	Best	Good	Reduce
Chilies	Best, dried	Avoid	Best
Cilantro	Good	Best	Avoid
Collard Greens	Best	Good	Avoid
Corn	Best	Good	Good
Cucumbers	Reduce	Best	Avoid
Dandelions	Best	Best	Avoid
Eggplant	Reduce	Good	Good if cooked
Endive	Best	Good	Reduce
Fennel	Good	Best	Good
Garlic	Best	Reduce	Best
Ginger	Good	Reduce	Good
Green Beans	Best	Good	Reduce, okay if cooked
Hot Peppers	Best	Reduce	Good
Jicama	Good	Best	Reduce unless cooked
Kale	Best	Best	Reduce unless cooked
Leeks	Good	Reduce	Good
Lettuce	Best	Best	Reduce
Mushrooms	Best	Good	Reduce

	SPRING	SUMMER	WINTER
Vegetables			
Mustard Greens	Best	Good	Reduce unless cooked
Okra	Reduce	Best	Good
Onions	Best	Reduce unless cooked	Good
Parsley	Best	Good	Good
Peas	Best	Good	Reduce unless cooked
Peas, Snow	Good	Good	Reduce
Potatoes	Good, baked	Best	Good, mashed
Pumpkins	Reduce	Good	Best
Seaweed	Good	Good	Good, cooked
Spinach	Best	Good in moderation	Reduce
Squash, Acorn	Reduce	Best	Good
Squash, Winter	Reduce	Good	Best
Sweet Potatoes	Reduce	Good	Best
Swiss Chard	Best	Good	Reduce
Radishes	Best	Reduce	Reduce
Tomatoes	Reduce	Good in moderation	Best
Turnips	Best	Reduce, except greens	Good
Watercress	Best	Best	Reduce
Zucchini	Reduce unless cooked	Best	Reduce unless cooked
Grains:			
Amaranth	Good	Reduce	Best
Barley	Good	Best	Reduce
Buckwheat	Good	Reduce	Good in moderation
Corn	Good	Reduce	Good in moderation
Millet	Good	Reduce	Good in moderation

	SPRING	SUMMER	WINTER
Grains			
Oats	Good, dry	Good	Best
Rice	Reduce	Best	Good
Rice, Brown	Good, long grain	Reduce	Best
Quinoa	Good	Reduce	Best
Rye	Good	Good	Good in moderation
Wheat	Reduce–Avoid	Good	Best
Legumes			
Adzuki	Good	Best	Reduce
Bean Sprouts	Best	Good	Reduce
Black Grams	Good	Best	Reduce
Favas	Good	Best	Reduce
Garbanzos	Good	Best	Reduce
Goyas	Best	Good	Reduce
Kidneys	Best	Good	Reduce
Lentils	Best	Good	Reduce
Limas	Best	Good	Reduce
Mungs	Best	Good	Good
Split Peas	Good	Best	Reduce
Tofu	Reduce	Best	Good
Nuts/Seeds			
Almonds	Avoid	Good	Best
Brazil Nuts	Avoid	Reduce	Best
Cashews	Avoid	Reduce	Best
Coconuts	Reduce	Best	Good
Filberts	Good	Reduce	Best
Flax	Avoid	Good	Best
Lotus Seed	Avoid	Best	Good
Macadamias	Avoid	Good	Best
Peanuts, raw	Avoid	Reduce	Best
Pecans	Avoid	Reduce	Best
Piñon	Good	Good	Best

	SPRING	SUMMER	WINTER
Nuts/Seeds			
Pistachios	Avoid	Reduce	Best
Pumpkin	Good	Best	Reduce
Sunflower	Good	Best	Good
Walnuts	Avoid	Reduce	Best
Dairy			
Butter	Reduce, eat before sunset	Good in moderation	Best
Buttermilk	Reduce	Reduce	Best
Cheeses	Reduce–Avoid	Good	Best
Cottage Cheese	Reduce	Good	Best
Cream	Reduce	Good	Best
Ghee	Good, reduce	Best	Best
Ice Cream	Avoid	Good	Reduce–Avoid
Kefir	Reduce	Reduce	Best
Milk	Avoid, or nonfat	Best	Good, not cold
Sour Cream	Reduce	Reduce	Good
Yogurt	Good in moderation	Reduce	Good
Rice/Soy Milk	Good	Best	Good
Meat and Fish			
Beef	Reduce	Good in moderation	Best
Chicken	Good	Good	Best
Crabs	Avoid	Good	Best
Duck	Good in moderation	Good in moderation	Best
Eggs	Good in moderation	Good	Best
Freshwater Fish	Good	Good	Best
Lamb	Good in moderation	Good in moderation	Best
Lobster	Avoid	Reduce	Best
Ocean Fish	Good in moderation	Reduce	Best

	SPRING	SUMMER	WINTER
Meat and Fish			
Oysters	Reduce	Reduce	Best
Pork	Avoid	Good	Best
Shrimp	Reduce	Good in moderation	Best
Turkey	Good	Good	Best
Venison	Reduce	Reduce	Best
Oils	*In general, reduce oils*		
Almond	Reduce	Good	Best
Avocado	Reduce	Good	Best
Canola	Good	Good	Best
Coconut	Reduce–Avoid	Best	Best
Corn	Best	Reduce	Good
Flax	Good	Good	Best
Mustard	Good	Reduce	Best
Olive	Reduce	Best	Best
Peanut	Avoid	Reduce	Best
Safflower	Good	Reduce	Best
Sesame	Reduce	Reduce	Best
Soy	Good	Best	Good
Sunflower	Good	Good	Good
Sweeteners			
Honey	Best	Reduce	Good
Maple Syrup	Good	Good	Best
Molasses	Good	Reduce	Best
Raw Sugar	Reduce	Good	Good
Rice Syrup	Reduce	Good	Best
White Sugar	Reduce	Reduce	Reduce
Condiments			
Carob	Good	Good	Good
Chocolate	Good or Reduce (depending on body type)	Reduce	Good

	SPRING	SUMMER	WINTER
Condiments			
Mayonnaise	Reduce	Good	Good
Pickles	Good	Reduce	Good
Salt	Reduce	Reduce	Best
Vinegar	Reduce	Reduce	Good
Beverages			
Alcohol	Reduce	Reduce	Reduce or Good (depending on body type)
Black Tea	Good	Reduce	Reduce
Coffee	Good	Reduce	Reduce
Sparkling Water	Good	Good or Reduce (depending on body type)	Reduce
Herb Teas			
Alfalfa	Good	Good	Reduce
Cardamom	Best	Reduce	Best
Chamomile	Reduce	Best	Best
Chicory	Best	Best	Reduce
Cinnamon	Best	Reduce	Best
Cloves	Best	Reduce	Best
Dandelion	Best	Best	Reduce
Ginger	Best	Reduce	Best
Hibiscus	Best	Best	Reduce
Mint	Reduce	Best	Good
Orange Peel	Best	Reduce	Best
Strawberry Leaf	Best	Best	Reduce
Spices			
Anise	Good	Good	Best
Asafoetida	Good	Good	Best
Basil	Good	Reduce	Best
Bay Leaf	Good	Reduce	Good
Black Pepper	Best	Reduce	Best
Chamomile	Good	Best	Good

	SPRING	SUMMER	WINTER
Spices			
Caraway	Good	Reduce	Good
Cardamom	Good	Reduce	Best
Cayenne	Best	Reduce	Good
Cinnamon	Good	Reduce	Best
Clove	Best	Reduce	Good
Coriander	Good	Best	Good
Cumin	Good	Good	Best
Dill	Good	Reduce	Good
Fennel	Good	Good	Best
Fenugreek	Good	Reduce	Good
Garlic	Good	Reduce	Good
Ginger	Good	Reduce	Best
Horseradish	Good	Reduce	Good
Marjoram	Good	Reduce	Good
Mustard	Good	Reduce	Good
Nutmeg	Good	Good or Reduce (depending on body type)	Good
Oregano	Good	Reduce	Good
Peppermint	Good	Good	Good
Poppy Seeds	Good	Reduce	Good
Rosemary	Good	Good or Reduce (depending on body type)	Good
Saffron	Good	Good	Best
Sage	Good	Reduce	Good
Spearmint	Good	Good	Good
Thyme	Good	Reduce	Good
Turmeric	Good	Good	Best

Now that you have a good idea of what foods to eat in each of the three seasons, let's take an extended look at a key part of the 3-Season Diet program, namely, when and how to eat. Eating the right food at the wrong time and in the wrong way is like runing on empty all day and then filling the tank after you put the car in the garage for the night.

CHAPTER 6

When to Eat and How to Eat: The French Paradox and the Midday Meal

ALL THE WHILE AMERICANS were struggling to excise every scrap of excess fat and cholesterol from their diets—and were growing fatter by the decade—the French were consuming gobs of butter and cream along with their steak au poivre and foie gras and pastries—and enjoying substantially lower rates of cardiovascular disease and serum cholesterol. How are we to make sense of this apparent paradox? What allows the French to eat all that great-tasting fat and sugar and enjoy a rate of heart disease 50 percent lower than our own? Some researchers have posited the healthful antioxidant properties of certain components of red wine, which the French consume in much larger quantities than Americans. That may be true, but it is only part of the answer. (The French, unfortunately, also suffer from a higher incidence of cirrhosis of the liver, but that's another issue.)

I believe that a large part of the French Paradox can be explained by the way in which French eating habits have tended to relieve stress, the leading cause of overweight. Throughout France, as in much of Spain, Italy, other Mediterranean countries, and much of the rest of the world, the big meal of the day is lunch. In France shops and businesses close and people gather for a midday meal that can take two hours or more, often accompanied by wine and followed by a brief siesta, and until recently many businesses shut down to allow uninterrupted time for a serious meal—even in busy cities like Paris. Large amounts of food, often rich in butter, oil, and other fats, not to mention dessert and coffee, are consumed at leisure, generally in family settings. Supper in these cultures is usually very light, consisting of little more than soup, salad, or other minimal fare. Our English word "supper" actually derives from the Old French word for "soup." (Playing off that association, I like to think of supper as a "supplemental" meal, rather than a major one. Even in the American South, they commonly call this meal "sup," short for their small supplemental meal.)

The net result of this seemingly hedonistic approach to eating is that the French receive the bulk of their required nutrients at a time when they can make use of them during the workday; one study has shown that they eat 60 percent of their food before 2:00 P.M. Digestion is aided by wine that also helps diners to relax, stimulated by coffee afterward, and enhanced by the leisurely setting. And the enormous satisfaction of an enjoyable meal eaten in such relaxing circumstances adds a level of pleasure that cannot fail to increase overall well-being. The traditional American Sunday dinner, eaten at great leisure in the early afternoon in several courses, often with wine and with extended family present, is no doubt a remnant of this agricultural-era repast. As I have already pointed out, when our ancestors worked long hours in the field, they made lunch the main meal of the day, and in agriculture-based societies such as France's, that model was retained even after people began working in factories and offices in the city.

It seems that as we lost touch with when to eat, we also forgot how to eat. One of my teachers in India told me of an old Vedic saying: "When you eat standing up, death looks over your shoulder." Imagine what they would say about eating while driving your car! The epitome of unconscious eating is a Weight Watchers promotion a few years ago that offered an "eat while you drive" breakfast kit. This particular bit of madness included a box that would hold the coffee and breakfast meal without spilling it all over your car, so you could drive with one hand while eating with the other, focusing fully on neither. We generally rush through our meals while driving, talking on the phone, opening mail, or even working at our desks, not focused on our food at all. No wonder we're always hungry—our bodies have little or no memory of having eaten anything!

Would the French style of eating work for people raised in America, though? After I had explained my system to a young woman who came to see me to lose weight, she gave me a surprised look and said, "My God! That's exactly what my dad did." Her father had suffered from high blood pressure and was overweight for years while living in the United States and consuming a typical American diet. When he retired, he and his wife moved to France, and within six months his blood pressure was normal and he had lost 30 pounds. The big secret behind his rediscovered health, he had explained happily to his daughter, was that he had started eating as the French do. He consumed large and relaxing meals at midday and found that his evening hunger was so dramatically reduced that he often had little more than soup for dinner. Another woman who was taking my program lit up when I came to the part about making the midday meal the main meal. She explained that her mom had just moved back in with her after having been diagnosed with high blood pressure as a result of putting on too much weight. Mom was a European immigrant who, after getting sick on the blood pressure medicine, decided to take matters into her own hands. She stopped her medication, stopped eating dinner, and went back to having the big, leisurely lunches she remembered from her childhood. In a few short months she lost 35 pounds and her blood pressure fell to an acceptable level.

À L'AMÉRICAINE

As a way of judging just how effective the French approach to eating has been in controlling weight despite the consumption of large amounts of fat, we have only to look at recent studies that examine changes taking place in France as their traditional mealtime begins to disappear. According to Dr. Eveline Eschwege, director of epidemiological research at the Institut National de la Santé et la Recherche Médicale in Paris (NSRM), the French equivalent of the National Institutes of Health, the French public is gradually but perceptibly gaining weight. Eight percent of French people now qualify as obese—although still well below the United States, which has an obesity rate of over 20 percent. Dr.

Eschwege lays the cause to the growing French imitation of Americans in everything, "including the way they eat." She cites an increase in the consumption of processed foods, sodas, and the American habit of eating all the time. She also notes the difference between the ingredients in traditional dishes and fast food. "There are no chemicals, no additives, in foods that go into traditional dishes like veal with cream sauce or roast chicken and vegetables," Dr. Eschwege says. "Also, traditional dishes like those are eaten at table, calmly, so that satisfaction is gained and no one is hungry two hours later."

An American journalist named Susan Herrmann Loomis, who has lived in France for ten years and visited regularly over the past twenty, also finds a big difference in French lunchtime habits, especially in medium to large cities, "where instead of the traditional hush as workers stop to eat, the sidewalks are filled with busy people, phones clapped to one ear as they munch a sandwich." Even more disturbing is a report from Dr. Marie-Françoise Rolland-Cachera at the NSRM that the rate of obesity among French children has tripled, from 3 percent in 1955 to above 10 percent in the late 1980s. Loomis notes that she has watched "French breakfasts gradually switch from bakery-fresh bread, butter, and coffee to packaged cereals and commercial hot chocolate." She has also seen potato and corn chips, which the French now affectionately call "sheeps," slip into the regular French diet, while packaged pizzas, hot dogs, and frozen dinners have become part of the national cuisine. Coca-Cola, she observes, is now "the drink most often offered to children at meals on special occasions, whereas even five years ago it was water, plain or with fruit syrup; in the old days, they drank wine. 'McDo,' or McDonald's, has become the destination of choice for many a family night out. A friend in Paris, a chef, recently told me about two Parisian children with full-time working parents who eat dinner every night at their neighborhood McDo."

What we see in these developments is that what is eaten may matter, but not entirely in terms of calories and fat grams. Processed food that is equal in calories and fat content to naturally prepared foods apparently has a greater capacity to pile on the pounds (and most fast food has a higher fat content than natural food). Moreover, food that is consumed under stressful circumstances—hurriedly, while driving, walking, talking on the telephone—is not digested and metabolized as efficiently as food eaten under more relaxed and leisurely circumstances.

I am frequently amazed at how the same food can affect the body totally differently based on how you eat it. Some years ago, before I had developed my current system of eating, I was preparing to work with three professional tennis players at my health center. While driving all over central Massachusetts trying to lock in a tennis facility where they could practice during their stay, I stopped at a pizza place and got two slices and a lemonade to eat in my car. When I got home around 4:00 P.M., I had to meet with a carpenter who was giving me an estimate about some work we were doing on our house. As I was walking him through the house, I suddenly felt so tired that I literally could not keep my eyes open. I had to fold my arms and prop up one of my eyes with my finger to keep it open as I tried to look and act intelligent—or at least awake. I don't remember ever being so tired in the middle of the day. At first I thought that it was the pizza, until I realized that we often had pizza as a staff lunch and I had never had this reaction. The difference with this meal was that I ate as I was driving and I don't think I digested one bit of it. It hit me like a rock, and my body was so overtaxed that two hours later I was asleep on my feet. The same meal eaten calmly while sitting down did not stress my digestion enough to knock me out in the afternoon.

STOP AND SMELL THE CARROTS

Digestion is a complex and interrelated process involving not only the alimentary canal but the senses as well. When you stick your fork into a piece of cooked carrot, lift it to your mouth, smell its odor wafting up at you, and savor its taste, its flavor sends a message to your brain through the senses. Your brain then relays the message to your stomach to let it know that carrots are coming and to release the appropriate enzymes and digestive juices. If you are racing through town in your car, talking on your cell phone, or watching the latest reports of murder and mayhem on the six o'clock news, that taste message from the carrot will never get to the stomach. All of a sudden the stomach looks up, sees carrots raining in, and yells, "Where did all these carrots come from?" It then goes into emergency or survival mode, sending all the wrong cues to the rest of the body!

Use your senses to help you slow down when you eat: Smell the food, enjoy its distinctive color and taste. This may be one area where we can learn from wine connoisseurs, who are often ridiculed for the attention they pay to the taste and aroma of fine wine, and the baffling array of terms they use to describe it. Watch people tasting wine at one of these sessions and you will see them swirl the wine in their glass, examine its color, and inhale its fragrance deeply several times before tasting the smallest drop, which they then savor and examine on their palates to determine the component elements of that particular wine. You can argue the health value of wine, but the stomach of a wine taster has no doubt exactly what to expect! Of course, I don't think a McDonald's meal could stand up to that kind of scrutiny. Savoring your food begins with eating something worth savoring; it may not have to be gourmet quality, but it should be wholesome and well prepared.

I believe the health benefits of slowing down and savoring one's food explain why in more traditional countries people often eat with their hands. In India, to eat with your hands is quite acceptable, and I typically did so when dining with my teacher on my many visits there. Once you get the hang of it, eating with your fingers provides an amazing contrast to Western-style dining. First of all, this makes it impossible to flip through a magazine, open your mail, or drive your car. If the phone rings, you let it go or let the machine answer, because you can't pick up the phone with food all over your hands! Eating this way, you are forced to focus on your food and nothing else. In America, sad to say, eating is just not enough stimulation all by itself, and people look for the distractions of reading magazines or watching TV to keep them company. Even animals seem to take their food more seriously than we do; if you disturb a dog while it's eating, it will growl or worse—even your own pet.

In this country, we think of eating with our fingers as something only children do—and maybe we can learn something from our kids in this arena. Observe young children eating when no adults are around and you will see that they do tend to eat with their hands, and maybe make a mess, but they also know when to stop eating and rarely finish the plates we have piled high with more food than they need. Instead of eating to satisfy our hunger, many in the West eat to satisfy the old dogma that if we don't finish everything on our plate we are wasting food as people elsewhere are starving. After one of my trips to India, I taught my four children how to eat with their hands as the people do there. I reminded them to eat mindfully and not just throw the food around and get it all over themselves, and they took to it naturally. Of course, I held these sessions in the privacy of my own home, never thinking of the social ramifications until one day when I took my wife and children out to a restaurant—something we didn't do very often when the kids were small. Without warning, they dug into their plates of spaghetti and sauce with their fingers! By the time I realized that spaghetti was not one of the foods we had practiced on so carefully, it was all over their shirts, to the vast amusement of everyone around us. I had to make a few adjustments to the hand-eating program after that. On occasion I still eat with my fingers myself, and without fail this slows down my mind so that I can stop thinking and begin eating.

FINDING THE TIME

Many people to whom I propose changing their eating habits offer the excuse that it is simply not possible for them to make lunch the big meal of the day, or to eat it under anything resembling leisurely circumstances. When I was addressing the Young President's Organization in Columbus, Ohio, a national group of men and women who owned their own million-dollar corporations before the age of 50, I made my usual pitch for eating a big, leisurely lunch. A bright, prosperous-looking executive raised his hand. "I have a business dinner almost every night of the week," he said. "How can I possibly follow this program?"

"How do you feel the next morning after one of those business dinners?" I asked.

He seemed surprised at the question. "I feel terrible," he said with a laugh. "And I don't drink, so I'm not hung over. I just feel logy, stiff, and fat, like I'm still trying to digest all that restaurant food."

I assumed that he could afford to eat in good restaurants, so the problem probably wasn't with the food itself but with having such a large meal so late at night. His body never had a chance to digest it all, and so when he woke up it was still very much with him. I then asked the group if the rest of them also had business dinners that forced them to eat late, and they all raised their hands. When I asked if they, too, felt terrible the morning after these large dinners, they once again agreed unanimously. It was no mystery to them that these big dinners were bad for them, but they had simply accepted that this was the price of being a prosperous executive in a competitive field. I suggested that their dinner partners, also in their forties, fifties, or sixties, probably suffered the same morning-after blahs.

"Most of the people in this room are executives with the power to make decisions," I said with a tone of challenge in my voice. "What if you were to decide that you wanted to conduct business in a way that actually made you and your colleagues feel better at the end of the day? Don't you think there's a good chance they would be thrilled to hold the next meeting over lunch rather than dinner?"

I pointed out that even if they stayed a little later at the office to make up for the extra time it takes to enjoy a leisurely lunch, they would still get home to their families a lot earlier than if they ate their business dinners out. Years ago when I was teaching in the Soviet Union, they had something called the "social program" after work. No business was discussed in the evening. We got together for a "sup," usually a soup or salad, and headed off to the ballet or symphony or to see the sights. Here in the West we just never stop working and eating.

I was certain that this one simple recommendation could strip the weight off their waistlines and add pounds of energy to their day, but I had to work hard to convince those young executives. During a recent seminar with the American Association of Retired People (AARP), I received an entirely different response. As I got to the part of my seminar about the importance of eating a big lunch and a light dinner, they all shrugged their shoulders as if to say, "What else is new?" When I questioned them, I discovered that my idea was no big deal for them because they had long ago figured it out. Since I usually meet a lot of resistance to this point and have to spend a great deal of time discussing the pros and cons of my approach, I was left scrambling for a way to fill time!

Funny how we often wait until it's almost too late to learn the lessons that have been staring us in the face for a lifetime. My wife's grandfather Momo (short for Mario) owned restaurants along the West Coast and had a big dinner probably every night of his adult life. But in his fifties he began to have intestinal problems, and as he got older he had to give up his late dinners and get to the restaurant before six. If I he ate any later than that, he would be up all night long with indigestion. As Momo got older he would say, "If you want to take me to dinner, get me there by five o'clock or don't take me." In later years he would need to get there by three or four or he could not eat. But why do we have to wait till we are 80 years old to figure out that we function better if we eat our main meal in the middle of the day?

I am sure you have noticed that most restaurants have their senior citizen's specials between 4:00 and 5:00 P.M. This is not so the rest of us won't have to watch the old folks eat, but because it is the only time they can digest dinner. When you get to be a certain age and are making up for a lifetime of abusing your body, you either do things the right way or you pay a price. Walk into any senior care facility and you will find that they all eat their main meal by 4:00 P.M., because if they eat later than that they are up all night—not watching a movie but suffering with gas and indigestion.

Of course, it isn't always practical to eat a large midday meal, but even if you can schedule your work around a big lunch several days a week you will feel the results. In chapter 9, I will describe some very practical ways to work what I call the big lunch into your daily routine. For now, I recommend proving the value of this program to yourself with a simple experiment. Have a typical large evening meal one night, and when you wake up the next morning, observe how you feel and write it down. Later that day, have a big lunch and light dinner, or no dinner at all, depending on your hunger, and the next morning write down how you feel and compare it to the previous day.

The simple medical truth behind this way of eating is that the digestive system is stronger and works more efficiently during daylight hours, the result of thousands of years of evolution during which humans have eaten this way. Although we are designed to digest and assimilate food better in the middle of the day, in our society lunch hour has become the time to do errands, grab a quick bite, and rush back to work, or simply eat at our desks, not missing a minute of precious work time. Yet if food is eaten in haste or followed immediately by vigorous activity, digestion and assimilation are impaired. We don't receive sufficient nourishment from our food and, consequently, a few hours later we feel hungry. That's why, around three or four in the afternoon, a lot of people feel a "sugar low" and head for the Coke machine, unwrap a Snickers bar, or slip out for a *latte mocha grande.* Unfortunately, over time these sugar-heavy, caffeine-infused snacks can sometimes trigger compulsive eating disorders.

Certain body types tend to be more susceptible to gaining weight, as we will see in chapter 7. When these types start restricting calories or forcing the body into a starvation state through some extreme diet, their bodies will, as we have seen, start to store fat and crave more sugar. Such dieters often start to purge themselves as a way to get rid of the food that they are starving for but know will make them gain weight—a clinical condition known as bulimia. They may even convince themselves to eat virtually nothing because they believe that all food is bad—the related condition known as anorexia nervosa. The longer they continue to starve themselves through either bulimia or anorexia, the more they drive their bodies to store what little food they do consume as fat. Powerful and debilitating psychological factors are clearly at work in these eating disorders and need to be treated, but the real key to remedying them is to convince the body that the emergency is over!

RICHARD'S STORY

A couple of years ago a man named Richard Barnes came to me weighing 408 pounds. "John, I've really got to lose this weight," he said. A commodities broker and good college athlete, he had been very active until quite recently, playing golf and softball. But his excessive weight was affecting his knees and joints, and he finally realized that it was both structurally dangerous and threatening to his general health. He was also having difficulty summoning the mental energy needed for his very demanding, high-stress job, and he sought me out in desperation.

I had a simple directive for Richard: "Eat only one meal a day, make it at noon, and make it huge and very relaxed. Have a Thanksgiving feast every day, and if you find yourself hungry at dinnertime, that means you didn't eat enough for lunch."

He looked at me as if I were crazy, but I repeated that if he felt hungry at night, it was because he didn't properly nourish himself at noon. I told him that what he ate, as long as it was balanced and healthy, was less important than how and when he ate it. By "when" I meant finishing the meal before 2:00 or 3:00 P.M. But I also encouraged Richard to drink copious amounts of water all day and to eat slowly and joyfully, focusing on his food as he ate it so that he would maximize his enjoyment. Teachers of mindfulness meditation sometimes use an exercise in which they have their students eat one raisin with completely focused attention—savoring its smell, its texture, the first explosion of flavor on the tongue and palate, the consistency of the raisin as they slowly chew it, and its lingering sweetness in the mouth and mind. They eat that raisin as if they were tasting a $500 bottle of aged Bordeaux! Imagine if you ate a whole meal of salad, vegetables, broiled fish, steamed rice, and dessert with that kind of focus. Do you think that two hours later you would have trouble remembering what you ate for lunch, as so many people do?

Most of us can't maintain that kind of awareness throughout an entire meal, and I didn't really expect Richard to do so. But I advised him not to distract himself by watching television, reading magazines, or talking on the phone. I told him to remember the golden rule: "Whatever the mind is doing, the body must do, and vice versa." If the mind is otherwise occupied while the body is trying to eat, then it will have no awareness of eating and will not even bother to send the proper signals to the salivary glands and digestive enzymes to do their jobs. The food, which is designed to nourish mind and body, will actually separate the mind from the body and the result will be either indigestion or lack of vitality.

After eating, to improve digestion, I suggested a 10-minute rest, lying on his left side, followed by a 5- or 10-minute walk. "Breakfast is optional," I told Richard. "If you need it, have it early and very light, preferably just some fruit." The old nutritional paradigm of building the day on a large, satisfying breakfast misses the point by several hours, because the body is not yet strong enough to digest a big meal; it is actually still in its elimination, or spring, stage between 6:00 and 10:00 A.M. Just as we don't eat heavy, protein-laden meals in spring, we should not put stress on our digestion by consuming an enormous breakfast before the body is ready to handle it. Nutritionist Adele Davis, who was very popular in the 1960s and '70s, used to advise people to eat breakfast like a king, lunch like a prince, and dinner like a pauper. She understood that we need big reserves of energy to get through the day, but her timing was just a little off. If you eat a big breakfast, you will not be hungry for lunch, and as a result you will definitely be starving for dinner and will be compelled to stuff yourself at a time when your body does not digest food with maximum efficiency.

Richard called me after the first week and said that he had not only lost 10 pounds but that he no longer felt hungry at night. In fact, he didn't feel hungry any time during the day, except perhaps just before lunchtime, when his appetite was primed for the big feast. "I have found myself eating late at night in front of the TV," he confessed, "but that was more out of habit than hunger." Once he became aware of his habitual behavior, it gradually ceased.

The next week he lost 3 pounds, then 7, then 10, for a total of 30 pounds in the first month. The second month he lost another 20, and after 3 months had lost a total of 68 pounds, without any dieting or strain. Although I restricted dinner for Richard because of his extreme overweight, even for someone without such a serious weight problem dinner is an optional meal, as I will describe in my weight-balancing program. If you do eat dinner, try to keep it light, because any food eaten after the sun goes down will be processed by a weaker digestive system. Once again, this regimen is intended for adults, who have stopped growing. Children still need to eat 3 times a day, as long as you serve them dinner before sunset.

SIESTA TIME

When I bring up the subject of eating a big lunch at my seminars, some invariably complain that when they do have a generous midday meal, they fall asleep at two in the afternoon. I tell them the same thing I will tell you: If you put gas in your car, you expect it to run, not stall out. By the same token, when we put fuel or food in our mouths we should feel an energy increase, not fatigue or depletion. The problem of sleeping after meals is related to whether you were rushed when you ate, the kind of food you ate, or the current state of your digestive system, not with the time of day.

During my studies in India, on many occasions I would eat with my teachers. One day while at a conference, we ate a huge midday meal that left me stuffed and ready for a nap. The conference hall was very hot, and the speakers spoke mainly Hindi, which I do not understand. I would often just sit there and try to look interested, occasionally getting a translation from one of the other doctors, or just reading. Sometimes a talk would be given in English, for which I was duly grateful. But on the whole I needed my utmost attention to stay focused on the lectures, and I well knew that if I went back in there after lunch I would immediately fall asleep. I told my teacher, Dr. Raju, that I was going to skip the afternoon lecture and go to my room for a nice, long nap.

"No," he said, "go to your room and lie on your left side for 15 minutes, a kind of siesta, and then I will come and get you. You will not fall asleep, and we will go to the hall together."

I told him I was sure to be asleep in five minutes, and if I did not answer the door to please go on without me. But I did what he said and sure enough, when he knocked 15 minutes later I was wide awake and feeling refreshed. The afternoon meeting lasting into the evening, and to my amazement I did not doze off once. "First of all," my teacher explained, "the food was well prepared, and although we ate a great deal, we ate the food slowly and calmly." This added to our satisfaction and greatly enhanced our digestion process. Dr. Raju also explained the secret of lying on your left side. Because of the asymmetrical shape of the stomach, lying on the left side allows the food to flow through it and into the small intestine. This is an old remedy for indigestion that has recently been documented by scientific studies showing that when people with heartburn and ulcers lay on their left side after meals, they did not need as much antacid medication as those who did not lie on their left side. This technique is particularly effective if you have eaten an extra-large meal and tend to fall asleep in the afternoon when you overeat.

The concept of the siesta in Mexico and southern European countries was not to doze through the entire afternoon, but to let the large meal be digested rather than racing back to work and compromising the digestive process. Rushing from a big meal into activity is the best way to get gas, feel sleepy, and be famished 3 hours later, because you never allow the nourishment to get into your bloodstream and provide energy. An appropriate siesta lasts 10 or 15 minutes after the large midday meal, preferably on the left side. If you are at a restaurant, you can lean to the left, and if driving your car make as many right turns as possible so as to push the food off to the left side. The important thing is to relax for 5 or 10 minutes after the main meal so that you can digest it efficiently and avoid the afternoon blues.

In a previous chapter, I discussed the case of Charlene, the emergency room nurse from Boulder who gained 105 pounds while dieting. While she was on my weight-balancing program, Charlene started taking a class in French cuisine. She would labor all morning, cooking a big feast, and then at midday, while her classmates carefully minimized their intake of the fatty, wonderful-tasting French cuisine they had prepared, from chicken with cream sauce to chocolate desserts, Charlene would eat her fill. Her classmates, who were all going home and having a regular American dinner in the evening complained that they were gaining weight. But by eating a large, relaxing, and very satisfying meal at midday, followed by a very light supper, in 1 year Charlene lost the 105 pounds she had gained while dieting.

When you eat your main meal at lunchtime, in a relaxed way with a little rest and a walk afterward, you can feast and still confidently engage in mental activity during the rest of the afternoon without getting tired. The net result will not only be more vibrant health, but also a gradual balancing of weight closer to your ideal level. As in all parts of my program, however, I do not want this suggestion to become stressful dogma. On those occasions when your family or friends are getting together for a celebratory dinner out, just eat a light lunch and enjoy your dinner. If you have been following my regimen with fair regularity, an occasional big dinner shouldn't cause you the gastric distress it otherwise might.

Another reason for eating your main meal early in the day may be even more important. The nervous system comes alive in midafternoon between 2:00 and 6:00 P.M., and it craves 80 percent of your daily ration of blood sugar. If all you have for lunch is yogurt or cottage cheese because you're "trying to lose weight" or "don't have time," then your system will go into survival mode. Your brain won't function fully, and your body will crave emergency fuel in the form of sugar and simple carbohydrates—sweets, sodas, salty chips, pizza, or coffee. Each time you binge on this emergency fuel, you will experience a fleeting burst of energy followed by an even stronger crash, and each emergency refueling will be less effective than the one before.

Worse even than eating foods that are antithetical to good nutrition, and sending the message to the body to store fat, is the *stress* that results from the body's response to low blood sugar. You have to ask yourself every day: Do I feel tired and sluggish in the afternoon? Do I crave emergency food after lunch? If the answer to either question is yes, then your eating habits are generating a survival response. The stress of that response causes your body to produce degenerative stress-fighting hormones and free radicals as waste products, which are disease producing. The good news is that if you can teach yourself to eat the kind of midday meal that will satisfy your nervous system's blood sugar needs, you will become energetically self-sufficient. You'll avoid that debilitating afternoon lull, you'll get rid of your cravings for sugar and caffeine, and you will succeed in convincing your body that your life is not an emergency.

LIFESTYLE TIP

Monitor yourself throughout the day. Check your energy and stress levels, particularly at the end of the day. Fine-tune your eating habits—how and when you eat—until you start to see stable energy all day long. Eventually you should have the same energy when you leave work as you had when you arrived.

CHAPTER 7

Fine-Tuning Your Diet According to Your Body Type

S O FAR WE HAVE seen that the three annual harvests translate into three principal seasons of the year, and that each of these seasonal harvests corresponds to a particular diet: low-fat in spring, high-carb in summer, and high-protein in winter. I often say that if we had no grocery stores or diet books and were forced to live off the land, we would eventually notice these things for ourselves. But we would also notice that not everybody on earth has the same kind of body. When we examine the classic body types closely, we find that many of them can be linked to ethnic origins from certain parts of the world. Over time these ethnic groups migrated and adapted to an environment that suited them perfectly. Mediterranean people, for example, have the ability to ingest more oils and live comfortably on fish, vegetables, and grains, whereas in the north, Scandinavians were forced to eat more meat and so need high-quality protein. Asians never drank milk; therefore most do not have the enzymes needed to break it down. Some people can live on raw fruits and vegetables, whereas others would wither away on such a diet. Thousands of years ago, before the various races and ethnic groups of the world started intermarrying, feeding each group was easy. People who could not tolerate the cold migrated to tropical climates and evolved smaller body types that could handle heat but were ill equipped to withstand the cold winters in, say, Norway or

Vermont. In the tropics, these types did well and nature supplied them with a perfect diet of lighter fruits and vegetables to feed their smaller and lighter constitutions.

Today many of the tropical types do live in Vermont, and if they ate a tropical diet of cold, light fruits and veggies they would freeze. Having some insight into your ethnic background through knowledge of your body type supplies an important piece of the nutritional puzzle. Even though many parts of the world remain ethnically intact—China and Africa, for instance—most of the world is rapidly becoming more diverse. People complain that diets that work for their closest friends and even extended family members don't work for them. Some have allergies to soy products or milk and others don't. Books have been written condemning or condoning certain foods based on only parts of the story. The truth is that intermarriage and migration over the past few centuries have not eradicated the impact of thousands of years of ethnic roots; today people with very different body types live not only in the same areas but often under the same roof, with many of their ethnic differences intact.

You have probably already noticed some of these differences yourself. We all know some people who tend to complain of cold hands and feet all year long, even in the summer. They embody nature's winter properties of coldness and dryness. Many of these so-called winter types migrate south to Florida and Arizona to stay warm. You may have also noticed that other people are more like summer. Their extremities seem to be so warm that they often don't wear coats, hats, or gloves in the wintertime. When I was growing up, everyone remarked that John F. Kennedy never wore a hat outdoors; he was a summer person who didn't need one. And then there are people who resemble spring. They're bigger boned and somewhat fresher and retain more water—just as the earth holds on to more water in the spring—so they may seem overweight, even if they are not. These spring folks often seem to have a runny nose and congestion and maybe a breathy voice, as if they suffered from allergies or mild asthma. (Think of Babe Ruth, for instance.) But aside from such observations, many of which you have probably made yourself, what is the significance of these different body types for our dietary needs and overall health?

Over the years, many different ways of categorizing body types, also known as metabolic types or constitutions, have been developed. Recently, for example, one prominent diet has been based on blood types, such as O or A negative, which ultimately derive from different ancestral, ethnic blood lines that indicate nutritional predispositions similar to those I discussed at the beginning of this chapter. Still other systems have been based on some combination of body size and proportions and basic temperaments. One of the most complete and fascinating such models was created by an American psychologist based entirely on personal observations. William H. Sheldon (1898–1977) taught and did research at several American universities and is best known for his series of books on the human constitution. According to a system he invented called "somatotyping" (from the Greek word for "body"), Sheldon classified people into three body types linked to certain personality traits and temperaments, using the terms "ectomorph," "mesomorph," and "endomorph." In Sheldon's classification, ectomorphs are generally tall and thin with a fragile frame and a large head—somewhat like our winter types who get cold very easily. They tend to be intellectual, verbal, and under stress may become scattered or nervous. Mesomorphs are classically athletic with a muscular, sturdy frame in the basic shape of an inverted triangle—broad shoulders and tapered waist. Born leaders, they resemble our hot, fiery, competitive summer types, who tend to be active and adventurous but who can sometimes be insensitive to the feelings of others. Endomorphs—who, like our spring types, have bigger, plumper bodies and are more sociable and easygoing—love food and comfort, but can often seem lethargic by comparison to the other two types.

Sheldon began his study of the human physique with photographs of 4,000 college men taken from the front, back, and side (he later went on to take tens of thousands of photos of men of all ages). By examining these photos he discovered that the three fundamental elements of body type were generally combined to some extent in all human bodies. Since virtually nobody represented only one type to the total exclusion of the other two, Sheldon worked out ways to measure these three components and to express them numerically so that everybody could be described in terms of three numbers ranging from 1 to 7, where 1 represents the minimum presence of a component and 7 the maximum. Someone who is predominantly mesomorphic but with a strong ectomorphic component and very little endomorphy, for example, Sheldon scored as 7-3-1. Going even deeper, Sheldon determined that the three basic somatotypes are related to different aspects of the body's biology. He held that endomorphy is centered on the abdomen and the digestive system; mesomorphy derives from the muscles and circulatory system; whereas ectomorphy is directly related to the brain and nervous system.

Sheldon's system works fairly well for understanding the relationship between body type and temperament, but it does not connect the constitutions either to nature or to any coherent system of nutrition and health. The system of medicine that I studied in India known as Ayurveda is thousands of years older than Sheldon's model and is derived from an in-depth study of nature itself. Ayurveda successfully integrates humankind and the natural world by linking body type to diet, temperament, environment, and many other interconnected factors that relate to health and well-being. The three basic body types that Sheldon called endomorphic, mesomorphic, and ectomorphic parallel nicely the three Ayurvedic body types known by their Sanskrit names of *kapha* ("earth, water"), *pitta* ("fire"), and *vata* ("air"), respectively. But I prefer to call the three types spring, summer, and winter, because they are in essence the three basic principles of nature that those Sanskrit words describe; I also believe they represent what Sheldon was on to. Everything in nature, including the earth, plants, animals, and people, is made up of unique combinations of those three basic principles. The precise amount of winter, summer, or spring qualities you receive at birth, determined to a large extent by your ethnic background, accounts for your individual constitution or body type. For example, someone who has a predominance of both summer and spring may be referred to as a summer-spring type, meaning a predominantly summer person who has certain springlike qualities as well.

Like Sheldon's system, the Indian model breaks down the body into three major components that we are always striving to keep in balance with each other: the musculoskeletal or structural system, the digestive system, and the central nervous system.

The body's structural system—muscle and bones—is heavy and solid, and holds on to water. Water and heaviness relate to spring, when the earth holds on to more water and grows heavier; hence the spring body type is bigger boned. These spring people are easygoing, calm, and slow moving, with slower metabolisms.

The digestive system is clearly a fiery system—the body's furnace digests and assimilates our food—and fire relates to summer. Summer people are themselves fiery, generally competitive, and highly energetic.

People with hypermetabolic, fast-moving constitutions belong to winter, when the nervous system is moving more quickly than anything else in the body—as quickly as the wind itself. In winter, the trees have shed their leaves so nothing stops the wind from blowing fast. That light, quick, windy quality relates to the nervous system. The downside of people with nervous energy is that their skin tends to dry out, their hands and feet get cold, and they suffer from joint irritations (as many people do during the winter season in response to the amount of winter in their constitution). The drier they get, the more their nervous system becomes agitated, and they often complain of insomnia and even worry and anxiety.

Just as each of three body types we've been discussing relates to one of the three harvest seasons, so our lives can be divided into three general periods, each of which reflects a particular season and related body type. In the earliest stage of existence, as a baby or young person, your skin is moist and resilient and your muscles are soft and flexible, because your system is flushed with water and liquidity in order to grow up quickly. We refer to this as the springtime of life, and it certainly does correspond to the spring season with its heightened moisture. As you move into the long middle period of life, your blood heats up and you become inflamed by the passions of sexuality, raising a family, work, competition, and the desire for material success, money, and power. You are susceptible to the same problems faced by summer types in summer—overheating and burnout. Finally, as you enter the latter part of your life, you begin to dry out and become more like winter—lighter, airier, less dense. Hence the classic migration for elderly people to the sunbelt states of Arizona and Florida. Many people even experience a change in their spiritual nature as they come closer to the end of life; their values and priorities often become less attached to the things of the material world and they begin to be more attentive to their spiritual needs.

We might summarize the seasonal course of life this way: The spring-like moisture of youth gives a baby the elasticity to grow like a weed; the heat of summer imbues adults with the fire needed to raise a family and make their stake in the world; and the drying winds of winter in old age stimulates the nervous system to find God and the meaning of life before it's too late!

Food, herbs, and medicines can also be classified according to their qualities of winter, summer, or spring. So, too, can animals: Look at a bear or an elephant, both of which are big and heavy and springlike. The tiger is fiery, aggressive, and competitive (summer type), whereas a mouse or deer is lighter, leaping and darting like the wind (winter type). If we look carefully, we can find the universal principles that underlie the 3-Season Diet at work throughout all of nature, including not only in the seasons but also at various times of day, in, and probably through-out the universe as well.

BODY TYPE VERSUS BODY IMAGE

Understanding body types can also help take some cultural pressure off those people who happen to have a constitution that is naturally some-what bigger and heavier than others. Looking at fashion magazines we could argue that in the United States, for instance, the most desirable body types for men and women these days are the waiflike winter types and athletic summer types, to the exclusion of bigger, heavier spring types. That's quite an irony since, especially among women, the most widely admired and desirable body type throughout the ages has been the spring type: big boned and voluptuous, with large breasts and hips, a wide face, thick hair, and big, wide-set eyes. These women radiate a maternal warmth and a calm, sweet demeanor that most people find irre-sistibly appealing. We see them in the paintings of Renaissance artists such as Titian and Rubens, whose women often seem gargantuan by modern standards, and more recently in the late paintings of Renoir and the sculptures of Gaston Lachaise, but the images themselves reach back to the goddess figurines that proliferated in Old Europe and the Middle East as much as 10,000 years ago. The women of the Renaissance may seem overly heavy to us, but excess body fat at a time when food short-ages were commonplace might have been be considered something of an insurance policy, not to mention a sign of wealth. And in India, where the seasonal system of body types was first codified, the big, voluptuous spring type was the undisputed preference conveyed in all the ancient texts.

When William Sheldon expanded his research into somatotypes in the 1950s to include women, he determined that women "are so much more endomorphic [springlike] than men that at all ages they are heav-ier in proportion to stature." The acceptable weight for most women in the 1940s and '50s was still somewhat higher than it is today. The aver-age Miss America weighed close to 140 pounds; voluptuous was in, and paragons of sexiness included the likes of Jayne Mansfield, Mamie Van Doren, and Marilyn Monroe. But in postwar America, a different trend began to take hold. The growing fashion industry, with the help of Madison Avenue's admen, was conspiring to convince women—and men—that women ought to aspire to the unrealistically slim and boyish figure of a fashion model, regardless of the fact that they are constitu-tionally heavier than men. Under normal circumstances, women have 22 percent body fat, compared to 14 percent for men, but now they were suddenly expected to have a body fat level closer to the male ideal—about 15 to 17 percent.

The burgeoning media in general, and television in particular, helped to universalize this unrealistic image of women based on fashion design-ers' idea of the perfect figure (or perhaps the figure that made their clothes look perfect). As a nation, it seems, we stopped listening to our own inner sense of what our bodies should be and heeded instead a body image imposed on us by fashion, the media, and Madison Avenue, whose job has always been to make us feel inadequate in order to sell us a product for our hair, our breath, our odor, our physique, or our weight.

This intense self-consciousness about physical image came at the very time when a booming postwar economy and advances in agricultural technology were making food more plentiful and more readily available than ever before. Even if the average American family couldn't yet afford a split-level home in the suburbs with two cars in the garage, they could afford to eat some form of meat every day—often two or three times a day—and not only meat but potatoes, gravy, and all the trimmings. Larger refrigerators and freezers made it possible to store plenty of meat, not to mention ice cream, waffles, and other highly caloric and processed food. In the face of such abundance, not overeating seemed downright un-American. And so a gradual tendency to overeat dovetailed with an increasingly unrealistic sense of body image to give Americans a complex about their weight. That led to obsessive dieting and has brought us to the dilemma in which we currently find ourselves.

IDENTIFYING YOUR BODY TYPE

Now let's take a look at the three basic constitutions and find some ways of determining which type or types fit you most closely. Think back to grade school and some of the characters you might have encountered among your classmates then. The winter type is epitomized by a young girl named Debbie. Compared to other girls her age, Debbie is slender and small boned and a little taller than most. With her long legs, she is also quite a bit quicker than her friends, but may also be a bit too inhibited to let her skills shine. Debbie is quick mentally, too, often getting the points the teacher is making before the rest of the class have caught on. That might explain why she frequently seems restless and easily bored, so much so that the teacher may have to ask her to settle down and be quiet.

Winter is characterized by cold and dryness, both exacerbated by the constant movement of the wind, and movement is precisely what predominates in Debbie's body type. She moves quickly, learns quickly, and also forgets quickly. Because her mind is constantly leaping from one thing to another, she has trouble focusing on one subject or project for any length of time. People sometimes refer to her pejoratively as "flighty." Debbie is one of those people I referred to at the beginning of the chapter whose hands and feet always seem cold, even in warm weather. Her hair is dark but has a tendency to be dry and brittle.

Debbie's classmate Kenny excels at schoolwork, particularly in more visually oriented subjects such as math and science. Redheaded and freckled, he is the classic summer type, strong, athletic, and fiery. He is extremely competitive and is quick to take command when necessary, either in class or on the playing field. His fiery mind tends to drive his body hard, and he tends to be a perfectionist. This trait makes him excel at whatever he chooses to do; on the negative side, it sometimes makes him too demanding of himself. If he doesn't win or come out on top it gets him down. By the same token, he can become impatient with classmates or even adults who don't match up with his high standards and expectations, and may speak or act insensitively. In the summer, Kenny's face turns bright red when he gets excited, which happens often because the summer body type carries a lot of heat by nature.

The third basic type, reflective of spring, is embodied in their classmate Tanya. One of the bigger girls in the class, Tanya is slow to learn, but once she "gets" something, she retains the knowledge for a long time. She is just the opposite of Debbie, who takes in information quickly but can't remember it for long. Tanya learns best kinesthetically, by doing things hands-on. But because most of her classes are taught visually with textbooks, videos, and blackboards, or auditorily, with lectures and discussions, she has a hard time in school. She excels in geometry and geography, however, which allow her to learn kinesthetically from shapes. Tanya is a late bloomer but eventually will be able to command any field of activity.

In terms of temperament, Tanya's demeanor is calm and tranquil, and she moves slowly and methodically, with no wasted effort. This ought to be a plus, but in our fast-paced society Tanya runs the risk of being labeled slow or even dyslexic, despite having as much natural talent and ability as the other types—perhaps even more. Tanya has great physical endurance and strength but is short on speed and agility. She would not make a world-class sprinter or rope climber, but her natural strength makes her popular when choosing up sides for soccer, and she would probably bat cleanup on the baseball team. Because of stress, diet, and lifestyle, Tanya can often complain of asthma, which may be induced by exercise. She has to watch her intake of certain mucus-producing foods or she will be unable to enjoy her physical abilities.

These three basic body types reflect the three fundamental governing principles of nature—winter, summer, and spring. At conception, we are all given some amount of each quality, and the proportion that we have—which qualities dominate our makeup—determines our overall type. Constitution is much more than just a body type, however; it is a true psychophysiological, temperamental, and mind-body type. Much more than just the size and shape of our bodies, it influences how we think, spend money, eat, and sleep.

CHARACTERISTICS OF THE WINTER TYPE
- Light, thinner build
- Performs activity quickly
- Tendency toward dry skin
- Aversion to cold weather
- Irregular hunger and digestion
- Quick to grasp new information, also quick to forget
- Tendency toward worry
- Tendency toward constipation
- Tendency toward light and interrupted sleep

CHARACTERISTICS OF THE SUMMER TYPE
- Moderate build
- Performs activity with medium speed
- Aversion to hot weather
- Prefers cold food and drinks
- Extreme hunger and quick digestion
- Can't skip meals
- Medium time to grasp new information
- Medium memory
- Tendency toward reddish hair and complexion, moles, freckles
- Good public speaker
- Tendency toward irritability and anger
- Enterprising and sharp in character

CHARACTERISTICS OF THE SPRING TYPE
- Solid, heavier build
- Greater strength and endurance
- Slow and methodical in activity
- Oily, smooth skin
- Slow digestion, mild hunger
- Tranquil, steady personality

- Slow to grasp new information, slow to forget
- Slow to become excited or irritated
- Sleep is heavy and long
- Hair is plentiful, thick, and wavy

Once you determine your body type, your unique combination of winter, summer, and spring, you will know your fundamental requirements for action in harmony with nature. Knowledge of your body type gives you an owner's manual, which includes your maintenance schedule and performance records. When you buy a car, you know you have to change the oil, so you want to find out exactly when to do that—every 3,500 miles or every 7,000. In the same way, knowing your constitutional type also involves common sense. If you're a hot person in a hot season, eat cool food. If you're cold and dry and feel like you're freezing all winter, don't eat raw vegetables just because you've heard that a raw food diet is good for your health. That kind of food might be good for some people some of the time, but it isn't going to be good for all of the people all of the time. Without such knowledge, you may enjoy optimal functioning, but it will be random. With it, you will have clear guidelines for which food is most suitable at a given time of year, how much exercise is good and how much may be harmful, when to exercise and when to rest. One simple way to hone in on your precise body type is to answer the questionnaire that follows.

BODY-TYPE QUESTIONNAIRE

This questionnaire contains five sections: Mental Profile, Behavioral Profile, Emotional Profile, Physical Profile, and Fitness Profile. Each profile is important to complete the picture of your constitution, and is divided into three columns for each of the primary types—winter, summer, and spring. For each item (sleep patterns, appetite, endurance, concentration ability, and so on), circle the answer that most accurately describes your long-term nature. If two answers apply, circle both. If none applies, leave it blank. Then tally each column. The column with the most marks is your primary type; the column with the second-largest number of marks is your secondary type. For example, if you score 15 winter, 24 summer, and 4 spring, your body type is summer-winter with a predominance of summer. If you score equally in all 3 categories, that means it is extremely important that you change your diet with each season. This type is like a high-performance race car. It requires a lot of maintenance but can outperform the other types.

Take the time now to fill out the questionnaire, and then we will analyze the results. If you have trouble answering the questions yourself, ask someone who has known you for a long time to fill out the questionnaire with you. How others perceive us is often quite different from how we perceive ourselves. *Note:* If this is a library book, please be kind to future readers and either keep your score on a separate sheet of paper or write so lightly in pencil that you can erase your marks after you tally your score.

MENTAL PROFILE

	WINTER	SUMMER	SPRING
Mental activity	quick mind, restless	sharp intellect, aggressive	calm, steady, stable
Memory	short-term best	good general memory	long-term best
Thoughts	constantly changing	fairly steady	steady
Concentration	short-term focus best	better than average mental concentration	focus for long time
Grasping power	quick grasp	medium grasp	slow grasp
Dreams	fearful, flying, running, jumping	anger, fiery, violent	water, clouds, relationships, romance
Sleep	interrupted, light	sound, medium	sound, heavy, long
Talk	fast, sometimes missing words	fast, sharp, clear-cut	slow, clear, sweet
Voice	high pitch	medium pitch	low pitch
Mental Subtotal			

continued on following pages

BEHAVIORAL PROFILE

	WINTER	SUMMER	SPRING
Eating	quickly	medium speed	slowly
Hunger	irregular	sharp, needs food	can easily miss meals
Food and drink	prefer warm	prefer cold	prefer dry and warm
Achieving goals	distracted	focused and driven	slow and steady
Donations	gives small amounts	gives nothing or large amounts infrequently	gives regularly and generously
Relationships	many casual	intense	long and deep
Sex drive	variable or low	moderate	strong
Works best	while supervised	alone	in groups
Weather	aversion to cold	aversion to hot	aversion to damp, cool
Reaction to stress	excites quickly	medium	slow to get excited
Financial	doesn't save spends quickly	saves but big spender	saves regularly accumulates wealth
Friendships	tends toward short-term friendships	tends to be a loner (friends related to occupation)	tends toward long-lasting friendships
Behavioral Subtotal			

EMOTIONAL PROFILE

	WINTER	SUMMER	SPRING
Moods	changes quickly	slowly changing	steady, nonchanging
Reacts to stress with	fear	anger	indifference
More sensitive to	own feelings	not sensitive	others' feelings
When threatened tends to	run	fight	make peace
Relations w/spouse	clingy	jealous	secure

	WINTER	SUMMER	SPRING
Expresses affection	with words	with gifts	with touch
When feeling hurt	cries	argues	withdraws
Emotional trauma causes	anxiety	denial	depression
Confidence level	timid	self-confident outwardly	inner confidence
Emotional Subtotal			

PHYSICAL PROFILE

	WINTER	SUMMER	SPRING
Hair amount	average	thinning	thick
Hair type	dry	medium	oily
Hair color	light brown	red/auburn	dark brown/black
Skin	dry/rough or both	soft/medium or both, oily	oily, moist, cool
Skin temperature	cold hands/feet	warm	cool
Complexion	darkish	pink–red	pale–white
Eyes	small	medium	large
Whites of eyes	blue or brown	yellow or red	glossy white
Size of teeth	very large or very small	small–medium	medium–large
Weight	thin, hard to gain	medium weight	heavy, easy to gain
Elimination	dry, hard, thin, constipation	many, soft to normal	heavy, slow thick, regular
Resting pulse			
Men	70–90	60–70	50–60
Women	80–100	70–80	60–70
Veins & tendons	very prominent	fairly prominent	well covered
Physical Subtotal			

FITNESS PROFILE

	WINTER	SUMMER	SPRING
Exercise tolerance	low	medium	high
Endurance	fair	good	excellent
Strength	fair	better than average	excellent
Speed	very good	good	not so fast
Competition	doesn't like competitive pressure	driven competitor	easily deals with competitive stress
Walking speed	fast	average	slow & steady
Muscle tone	lean, low body fat	medium w/good definition	bulk w/higher fat percentage
Runs like	deer	tiger	bear
Body size	small frame, lean or long	medium frame	large frame, fleshy
Reaction time	quick	average	slow
Fitness Subtotal			

TOTALS

	WINTER	SUMMER	SPRING
Mental			
Behavioral			
Emotional			
Physical			
Fitness			
Mind-Body Type			

BRINGING IT ALL BACK HOME—APPLYING BODY TYPE TO YOUR DIET

Now that you've determined your dominant body type, let's look at some examples of how constitutions–yours and other people's–affect eating patterns. Summer types don't like hot weather, for example, and prefer cold food and drinks, especially in summer. But because of the fire in their constitution, they metabolize food quickly and tend to need refueling more than other types, and so they often suffer very intense hunger pangs and tend to get both light headed and short tempered when they need to eat. If your boss is a fiery summer type, don't go asking for a raise at eleven-thirty in the morning, just before lunch. Wait until your boss eats lunch and comes back feeling fueled up; then you can ask for anything and you'll get a much better reception. Even if the answer is no, it will likely be delivered with more good humor. Since summer types are prone to anger, you have to learn to pick your spots with them. They also tend to be good speakers and good competitors, but when they get out of whack, their disturbances may manifest as various forms of heat: rashes, inflammations, peptic ulcers, heartburn, poor vision, excessive body heat, and excessive perspiration, or as emotional states such as hostility or irritability.

I mentioned that spring body types have fallen out of favor in America. What makes life even more difficult for them is that the American diet favors mainly sweet, sour, and salty foods, all of which aggravate spring qualities because they tend to build up and hold on to water. The net result is that people with spring constitutions often gain weight out of proportion to how much they actually eat. They need to pay even more attention than the other two types to the spring antidote diet described in chapter 4.

Winter types suffer from a different kind of imbalance. Because their metabolism moves so quickly and their nervous system is going so fast, they lose their internal "eye of the hurricane" very easily. They tend to have no solid routine to their lives, eating here and there, on the run. What they need more than anything else is to lock in some good habits, which is what the 3-Season Diet with its big midday meal will do for them. They're still going to be free-flowing, fast-moving, creative, even off-the-wall people, but they will have some welcome stability to help keep them from falling into anxiety, worry, or depression. Winter types also need to follow the seasonal diet because when they get out of balance, they may develop dry skin, insomnia, constipation, fatigue, tension headaches, and arthritis. And because they burn everything off so fast, they can become underweight.

The "grazing" diet that I discussed in chapter 2 has become so popular largely because the winter style of functioning is increasingly prevalent in America: fast paced, always moving, always thinking. A recent diet article in *Reader's Digest* recommends the best way to combat stress: Eat small meals at frequent intervals so your stomach won't have to digest too much food at one time! Besides, most people want to eat every two hours to keep their energy up anyway. That may work for a while for genuine winter types, but even for them it will eventually decondition their ability to digest a big meal and make energy last, which was never their strong point to begin with. So it's important for winter types to realize that even though they can get away with eating frequent, small meals for a time, if they don't eat at least one serious midday meal each day they will run out of energy over the long haul.

If you are a winter type, you had better be extra careful to eat plenty of proteins and fats and oils and maximize warmth and moisture during those winter months—because the extent to which you get dried out and cold in the winter is the extent to which your body will make mucus in the spring. If you don't eat bitter greens in the spring to help the liver detoxify and cool your blood, then when the summer heat comes it will very likely overheat your body and compromise the liver's ability to do its job. And if you have a hot body going into the hot summer months, and you're a hot constitution to boot, you'll be in trouble. Like a desert, you will dry out. If you end the summer overheated and dry, the dryness of winter will further dry out your body. Come spring, the mucus membranes in your sinuses and intestines will be so dry and irritated that they will make even more mucus as a response to the dryness. When the mucus membranes become too dry or too wet, they lose their immune-protecting properties and become susceptible to infections, bacteria growth, and yeast proliferation.

You should also try to be aware not only of your body type and the season but of where you are geographically at any given time. One patient in her early fifties named Marjorie came to see me complaining of hot flashes. After reading a book on women's health, she wanted to find an alternative to hormone replacement therapy, which wasn't working for her. Within 4 months I was able to get Marjorie off all her hormones with a nutritional program consisting of specific herbs that act as natural hormonal precursors to estrogen and progesterone. Then she went on vacation to Hawaii for 2 months. About halfway through her vacation, Marjorie called to tell me that her hot flashes were starting to come back slightly. I advised her to increase her herbs, but 2 weeks later I got another call from her telling me that she was still having the flashes. Her vacation was almost over by then, so I asked her to come see me as soon as she returned home.

When I saw Marjorie again, it was apparent that she was overheated from the weather in Hawaii. I suggested that she eat an extreme summer antidote diet (see page 84), including extra aloe vera to help cool her down, and within a couple of weeks her hot flashes were under control again. I had never seen this relationship between hot flashes and a hot environment before, but it made sense. Marjorie was a summer body type staying in a tropical climate for an extended period, and complaining of too much heat in her body! The foods in the summer antidote diet cooled her down enough, along with the herbal support, to keep her hot flashes at bay. Food can often be your best medicine, and when you are eating in harmony with the seasons, beneficial foods will naturally become your preference.

All the factors of body type, season, climate, and geography add up. To avoid negative consequences, we have to eat the foods that nature provides as an antidote to these conditions. I believe that if we ate this way from birth, as nature intended, we could easily live past 100 and still be vibrant and youthful. We have the agricultural resources to make that a reality; we just have to learn to use them properly.

BODY TYPE AND ETHNIC ROOTS

Although arguments abound over how the different constitutions developed initially, I believe that they ultimately derive from where one's ancestors lived, and are based on the expression of nature in that part of the world. Because the first humans emerged in a warm, tropical environment, they developed small-framed, cool winter body types as an antidote to the heat. Nature is always a balancing act. If you live in a warm place, nature will provide a naturally cooling diet and a cool body type as a defense against the heat. If you then migrate to a cold environment, you will develop a warm body type. Think, for example, of Ireland, Scotland, and northern England, where the climate is wet and cold. People there tend to be light skinned, red complected, and medium framed and are known for their fiery tempers and personalities. As a whole they seem to have more of the summer qualities necessary to combat the cold, windy, and wet conditions on the northern European coast. Their body types have adapted over the millennia to the climate in which they live. Then think of tropical areas such as Mexico, Puerto Rico, and Cuba, where the weather is hot. The native peoples there are generally small framed and do not like the cold. Much like the earliest humans, they have winter body types perfectly suited to a hot environment. In contrast, the the bigger-boned Vikings who inhabited a place like Scandinavia, which has a cold but very dry climate, developed a heavier body type that was better insulated against the cold and dry climate. They had to survive by eating more meat than their ancestors in the tropics, because that was all they had to eat for much of the year; over time their high intake of meat and fish gave them more insulation and body size than was needed by the winter types in the Caribbean.

Although the geographic and ethnic origins of people play an important role in determining their body type, so does the climate in which they currently live. This is particularly clear when we look at the way America's earliest immigrants developed based on whether they took up residence in the North or the South. Beginning in the 17th century, people in the the American South, where the environment is very humid and damp, developed distinctly different behavioral characteristics from their Northern counterparts. Southerners typically appear easy going and calm, even lethargic by Northern standards, where the air is colder and drier most of the year and people move at a far brisker pace. As a group, Southerners seem to be more dominated by spring, and Northerners by winter—yet both groups originally shared the same geographic and ethnic identity, having emigrated mainly from England, Ireland, and Scotland. Descendants of a family that immigrated to Atlanta or Baton Rouge will have different body types today than their relatives whose forebears settled in Boston or New York. People who live in the North, yet have winter body types, are likely to complain that it's too cold, and they would like to live in the South.

Food also plays a role in all this. It's no accident that grains indigenous to the South tend to be dry, like corn, which is the driest grain of all. Southerners eat hominy grits because the corn from which grits are made helps dry them out and break up all the mucus, as do the fiery spices common in, say, Cajun and Mexican cuisine. (Although the U.S. "corn belt" now comprises Iowa and Illinois, corn is actually indigenous to Mexico, where it was originally harvested before the late winter monsoons, to be eaten in the wettest time of year there. For more detailed information on the origins and uses of corn and most other foods, please consult the Glossary of Foods, Appendix 1.) In the North, the most common grain is wheat, whose high gluten content and mucus-producing properties are needed to offset the cold, dry climate of winter. In terms of climate and geography, the same kind of north-south dichotomy is generally apparent in Europe and Asia, and in reverse in the Southern Hemisphere. (For example, the pace of life in Rio de Janeiro, São Paulo, and Buenos Aires in southern South America is faster moving and less tropical than the Amazon rain forest of northern Brazil.)

We cannot effectively make these generalizations for every culture on earth, because in the last thousand years humanity has changed dramatically through a combination of migration, invasions, and intermarriage. But the underlying qualities are clear in each of us if we look closely enough. I like to think of body type as a way of fine-tuning the 3-Season Diet to adjust for the fact that many ethnic groups now live together. In a world melting pot, you also need to look at who you are as an individual. Once you know how much winter, summer, and spring you have in your constitution, you can make slight adjustments in the basic 3-Season Diet to suit your needs based on your body type and certain other determinants. You can discern your strong points and weak points, and what you need the most and what the least. If you have a lot of summer, for instance, and you're heading into the summer season, whether it be in Boston, Florida, or California, you would simply follow the summer diet more strictly, since it is rich in cooling foods that will help to keep your summer constitution from getting overheated.

Let's say you are a winter type with Caribbean roots and tend to get very cold in the winter—but you live in New York City. During the cold winters there, it is important not only to follow the winter antidote diet to the letter, but also to start it a bit early, perhaps in the beginning of October instead of November, and continue it through April instead of March. This is just one more way to help your body type cope with the tension between your inherited body type and the geography where you live. Your diet will be your best medicine for preventing any imbalances. So although a winter type may not do as well in New York in the winter as a summer type would, if you adjust your diet you will do just fine. Here are some general guidelines that will help you make the necessary adjustments to your diet based on your type. Just keep in mind that nature's 3-Season Diet will provide balance for all three types in each of the three growing seasons. The body type recommendations that follow are intended only to help you fine-tune this diet.

BODY TYPE	RECOMMENDATION
Winter	Extend winter diet
Summer	Extend summer diet
Spring	Extend spring diet

If you are a combination type such as winter-spring or summer-winter, it is not necessary to extend the diet and make that season longer. You should merely follow the appropriate diet more strictly during the season that matches your type. For example, if you are a winter-summer type, your primary focus should be on the winter antidote diet, with secondary focus on the summer antidote diet. During the spring you should still follow the spring antidote diet, only not as intensely, or only intensely for 4 to 6 weeks instead of 4 months (as you would if you were a spring body type). If you are a spring-summer type, you will have to be stricter on the spring antidote diet and fairly strict on the summer antidote diet. You don't have to be as strict in the winter, but you should still shop from the winter grocery list. Following these diets is easy if you use the grocery lists in Appendix 3. Chances are your family will never know the difference when they eat according to the seasons.

CHAPTER 8

The Daily Cycle

A S WE HAVE SEEN, nature thrives on cycles based on its own internal rhythms, such as the annual cycle of the seasons and the harvests. The more we understand these rhythms and the more closely we can align ourselves with them, the easier our lives will be. In chapter 6, I explained some of the compelling reasons for eating your biggest meal in the middle of the day. But there's another reason that fits right in with my discussion of the links between the seasons and our constitutions.

Every creature within nature, including human beings, operates according to what are known as diurnal or circadian rhythms—patterns of physiological functioning that repeat every 24 hours. Birds wake up with the sun and go to sleep when it sets. Some flowers open their petals in the daylight and close them again at dusk. In humans, specific biochemical patterns recur regularly and predictably, day after day. For example, cortisol, a stress-fighting hormone produced by the body and released into the bloodstream to help cope with the stress of daily life, increases in the early morning hours and decreases in the evening. When we sleep, blood pressure, heart rate, and body temperature drop, then rise again in the morning. We are intimately connected to the daily rhythms of Mother Nature. The invention of the electric light about a century ago has helped to disconnect us from those rhythms, and has required still other inventions, like the alarm clock and the sleeping pill, to counteract that disconnection.

When we observe nature, we find that the same cycles we see in the seasons appear in microcosm in the course of a single day. These cycles mimic the three seasons once in each 12-hour period, as follows:

Spring	6:00 A.M.–10:00 A.M.	Muscles get stronger
Summer	10:00 A.M.–2:00 P.M.	Digestion stronger
Winter	2:00 P.M.–6:00 P.M.	Nervous system activates
Spring	6:00 P.M.–10:00 P.M.	Metabolism lowers for sleep
Summer	10:00 P.M.–2:00 A.M.	Liver is activated for cleansing
Winter	2:00 A.M.–6:00 A.M.	Cortisol levels increase

In summer, when the days are long and the nights are short, these time slots will be extended somewhat during the daylight hours and shortened in the evening. In the winter it is just the opposite. In other words, these times are based more on sunrise and sunset than on the hands of the clock, so adjust accordingly.

Just as it's better for us to eat certain foods during each season, we are also better off performing certain activities during different times in the daily cycle. Have you ever noticed that if you wake up in the morning and then go back to sleep, you feel sluggish much of the day? Yet if you get out of bed before 6:00 A.M. and start your day, you're more likely to be energized and upbeat all day (assuming you got enough sleep the night before). That's because the time of day that precedes sunrise shares the characteristics of the winter body type—lightness and quickness, for instance. When you arise during this time you naturally take on those characteristics. The very early morning between 2:00 and 6:00 A.M. is also the time believed to be most conducive to prayer and meditation in many spiritual traditions, both Eastern and Western. Earlier I said that as people enter the winter stage of their lives overall, they often tend to become more spiritual, which is another way of saying they grow lighter and less attached to material things. The same is true of this winter time of day.

But once you enter the spring cycle at sunrise, from about 6:00 to 10:00 A.M., your body naturally becomes heavier—like the spring body type. If you haven't already awakened and started your day, you're more likely to get bogged down with the heavy, lethargic feelings of this time in the daily cycle.

I once had a patient from Washington, D.C., who had woken up with a splitting headache every day for as long as he could remember. He came to me as a last resort after failing to get help from other doctors. I tried a variety of herbal treatments with no success. Then during one visit I asked him what time he usually woke up in the morning, and he told me around 10:00 A.M. When I asked when he went to bed, he said 1:00 or 2:00 A.M. I suggested that, as an experiment, he try to get to bed around 10:00 P.M. for 1 week and see if he could get up and out of bed before the sun rose. Although he was reluctant to change his routine so radically, he agreed to give it a go for 1 week. He followed my suggestion to read a boring book at around 8:00 P.M. (not my book, of course), and see if that would help him fall off to sleep. The very first night the gambit worked, and he woke up that next morning with no headache. Incredulous, he tried it for the rest of the week with the same result, and from that day on he was headache-free.

I explained to my patient that when we consistently wake up after sunrise, the body holds onto more of the heaviness of morning, which then accumulates in the body during the day and can lead to lethargy, dullness, and other physical ailments. To counteract the heaviness of the spring in this time of morning, the best antidote is physical exercise. The facts support this insight, since the majority of people who exercise regularly do it in the morning, often before starting their workday. Studies have shown that 75 percent of Americans who have a morning exercise routine are still working out a year later, as opposed to only 25 percent of those who exercise on their lunch hour or after work. Any kind of physical activity can help you at this time, whether it's gardening, walking the dog, or cleaning the house. In agricultural societies, this is often the time to plow the fields, when the muscles are strong and their heavy, springlike shock absorption qualities can stand the physical labor best. But since this heavy labor must get done before the sun grows too hot, on the farm the day starts early. As in the spring season when the body is forced to burn fat, this is the time of day to mobilize your fat cells. So long as the work is not done in a panic and you breathe properly (as we will see in chapter 10), you will force the body into fat metabolism each day. If you fail to get your metabolism up in the first part of the day, the body will stay sluggish all day, leaving the fat stored and heavy. As this fat accumulates over many years, you may have more difficulty getting up and moving through the early morning blahs, and if you don't get those fat cells burning in the morning, chances are you will burn sugar and store fat for the rest of the day. In chapter 10 I will show you some simple fat-burning exercises to start your day off right.

In nature, the norm is to wake up with the sun and watch it rise, although few of us who don't live on a farm ever do this anymore. We wake up with the jolt of alarm clocks or clock radios (nothing like the morning news, filled with mayhem, to start your day), and coffee to rev up our sluggish engines. The later you go to bed, the less likely you will be to see that sun rise—and every minute you lie in bed after the sun rises, you accumulate more heaviness and stiffness, and the longer it will stay with you during the day. Years ago, Soviet researchers also determined that the muscles are actually strongest from 6:00 to 10:00 A.M., and structured many of their weight-lifting competitions in the mornings for this reason.

I often ask my patients how they would feel if they went to bed at midnight and woke up at 10:00 A.M. They usually answer that they would feel groggy, stiff, and dull. Then I ask them how they would feel if they went to bed at 8:00 P.M. and woke up at 6:00 A.M. They instinctively answer that they would probably feel chipper. I then have to point out that in both instances they would have slept the same amount of time—10 hours—and the only difference was when they got the sleep. The same principle applies not only for sleeping but for eating as well. When we follow nature's rhythms, we invariably end up merrily rowing downstream—and when we do that, life really *is* a dream.

The hottest part of the day, when the sun is climbing to its zenith, is clearly the summer time of day. The digestive fires are being kindled and, as we have already seen, this is the ideal time to consume a meal large enough to provide fuel for the rest of the day and still be easily digested. This is not the best time for vigorous exercise; your midday meal should be followed by 5 or 10 minutes of rest, if possible lying on your left side, which supports better and more efficient digestion. If time still permits, you may then take a 5- or 10-minute walk.

If you've had the kind of large, leisurely lunch I have advocated, your body will be primed to work through the rest of the afternoon. Since winter is related to the activity of the nervous system, the 4-hour period that follows lunch, from 2:00 to 6:00 P.M., is the appropriate time for heavy mental activity and not as much physical labor. The brain uses about 80 percent of the body's glycogen, or energy supplies, during this time, so if you're feeling sleepy or listless or craving emergency fuel during the afternoon, it's probably because you ate too *little*, rather than too much at lunchtime—or you raced through that meal while driving, reading, working, or watching television.

During the four hours following "sunset" from 6:00 to 10:00 P.M. (the actual time of sunset will vary with the seasons, of course), the body reverts to spring mode. This marks the start of the second 12-hour cycle and is the second-best time to do physical exercise. If you've had a good-size lunch, you should be able to work out without stopping for supper, or after a very light meal. But the second cycle of the day is designed by nature not to enter into more vigorous activity but to begin to rest and relax because the body is gearing down for sleep. After the sun sets, digestion and cortisol levels go down, making it very difficult to digest a large dinner. It's natural to start feeling a bit lethargic or even sleepy midway through this second spring period.

Some of us are convinced that we are nocturnal—"night people" or "night crawlers"—and that it's natural for us to come alive after dark. But based on observations of our internal circadian rhythms, the rise and fall of our body temperatures, the increase and decrease of cortisol levels, and many other bodily adjustments that take place in the course of a 24-hour cycle, we know that human beings are not nocturnal. The idea of being a night person makes for a nice romantic fantasy, and it may even work when we're young enough to overcome the deficits of a big night out. But if you honestly observe yourself for a few nights between, say, 7:00 and 9:00 P.M., you will probably notice a pleasant drowsiness come over you. That's the time to give in to your body's natural rhythms and get to bed, as early as it may seem. Ironically, if you eat a big dinner during the 6:00 to 10:00 P.M. period, it may well keep you up late, as your body struggles to digest it. You may feel too full and bloated to relax enough for sleep.

Unfortunately, we have been conditioned to make ourselves stay up—to have a "nightcap" or a late-night snack, or watch a late movie. Now, of course, movies (and just about every other kind of programming) are on 24 hours a day. And the fact is that if you force yourself to stay up past 10:00 P.M., you may very well get a burst of energy that will propel you into the wee hours. The span of time between 10:00 P.M. and 2:00 A.M. is the second summer period of the day, and like the first, your digestive fires will come alive if you're awake. You may be able to work and you may also get pretty hungry and enjoy a substantial late night snack. But you will pay the price the next morning, when you will feel sluggish and heavy because your body has been on the night shift trying to digest that big meal.

During that second summer period of the day, the body moves into a liver-cleansing cycle. Studies have shown that the antioxidant glutathione peroxidase in the liver becomes active around this time and begins to detoxify the liver and the blood. Think of the janitor of a large office building who comes in at night to clean the floors and windows and empty the trash baskets while the offices are quiet. Then imagine what would happen if those offices were going full blast all night; the janitor wouldn't be able to do his job very well, and he might have to tell you he'll come back tomorrow. The purpose of our second summer period is to increase metabolic activity during the night to clean the blood and repair damaged tissue. If you are up, wired for sound, and having midnight snacks, the body's energy gets diverted to outward activities, and you miss out on this crucial internal cleansing time. This is no big deal once in a while, but if you keep turning the janitor away, pretty soon the office is a mess and you can't get any work done. If your body's resources are being used on a regular basis for eating or partying when the cleanup crew is supposed to be on the job, the body begins to push its impurities back into the bloodstream. Then it's only a matter of time before the body breaks down. And if you are living against the grain of nature for 10 or 20 years, the degenerative effects only multiply.

Even if you do get to bed early, the internal cleansing energy may still not be available for cleanup and repair if the evening meal was large. If the body has a difficult time digesting food, the energy that was slotted for maintenance is used for digestion. This digestive energy is often too little, too late, anyway, because the food has already sat there for 2 to 3 hours and normal digestion and assimilation are impossible. Then not only do you have undigested food wreaking havoc and being stored as fat in the body, but your internal cleansing cycle is also compromised. That's why many people wake up feeling so stiff and groggy. They say that what you eat at night you wear first thing in the morning. The old saying "Early to bed and early to rise makes you healthy, wealthy, and wise" was drawn from thousands of years of living in harmony with nature. Traditionally, we lived much closer to the land and respected the cycles of nature as a great boon rather than an imposition. The Native American have a saying of their own: "Always go to bed two hours after the sun sets"—which means changing with the seasons. Bedtimes and mealtimes would naturally be earlier in the winter, allowing us to get more rest, and later in the summer as the days get longer. By storing up rest in winter along with proteins and fats, we have the energy to make it through the long days of summer that call for the expenditure of tremendous amounts of energy. Most people do this naturally but do not even realize it. It's easy to go to bed early in the winter (when the sun sets at 5:00 P.M.) and sleep almost until the sun rises at 7:00 A.M. In the summer, when the sun stays up much longer and rises much earlier, the sleep cycle naturally shortens. I'm told that in Alaska the locals tend to sleep virtually all winter and stay up all summer. On the equator, where the days are always the same length, nature provides a harvest that is loaded with more high-carb or high-energy foods. Many more summer antidote foods are harvested and available naturally to offset the longer and hotter days there, compared to the Northern or Southern Hemispheres.

LIFESTYLE TIP

T RY THIS ROUTINE for 1 week and experience what it is like to paddle downstream for a change. Pick a week that is free of evening activities. When you wake up on the first day, roll out of bed and do some of the stretching exercises in chapter 9. If you have time, try to get outside for a 10-minute walk or jog, whichever you can handle. Be sure to breathe as I will explain in chapter 10. This 10-minute morning jaunt will force the body into fat metabolism and stabilize the blood sugars for the whole day, assuming you eat right. So eat a light breakfast and between noon and 3:00 P.M. try to stop and eat your largest meal of the day. Don't race through it, and rest and relax for 10 minutes after that meal. Monitor your brain's performance in the afternoon, and watch for any cravings.

In the evening have a light supper and around 7:00 or 8:00 P.M. take out a boring or relaxing book (this is not the time for page-turners). If all goes well, you will notice a natural sleepiness between 8:00 and 10:00 P.M.; give in to it and go to sleep. Around 5:00 or 6:00 A.M., you may wake up spontaneously and see by the clock that you have more time to sleep in. The first couple of days, go ahead and sleep in. But if you have been doing the daily routine I have laid out, by the third or fourth day your eyes will open at 5:00 or 6:00 A.M. and you will have enough energy to get out of bed and feel the lightness nature intended you to start your days with. Soon you will get accustomed to feeling fresh without morning stiffness, and it will become the way you prefer to live your life. If you have ever gone camping, you have probably experienced this naturally. You were in bed shortly after sunset and up with or before the sunrise. Just because we live in a house does not mean we have to insulate ourselves from the life-supporting cycles of nature.

At the end of this 1-week trial, I hope you will find it hard to turn your boat back around and start paddling upstream once again!

The
Complete
Weight-
Balancing
Program

PART II

CHAPTER 9

The Weight-Balancing Program

A T ONE OF MY recent seminars I was introduced to a 55-year-old man named George. After many years of frustration with just about every weight program available, George had seen an ad in the paper for my weight-loss and fitness seminar and, with a great deal of skepticism, signed up for my class. For the last 15 years he had been struggling with what he referred to as "creeping weight gain." He was about 40 pounds overweight, and in an effort to reverse the bulge for both health and vanity reasons, he had tried just about everything: macrobiotics, raw food and juice diets, health spas, fasting, exercise with personal trainers, even herbal wraps. Along the way he had also followed a number of the best-selling diets on the market. Despite all his efforts, George's weight kept increasing and he grew exasperated by all the conflicting advice he was getting: "Eat more, eat less, eat meat, reduce protein, be a vegetarian, avoid carbohydrates, exercise more."

After starting the weight-balancing program at my workshop, however, George reported that he lost 10 pounds effortlessly in 2 weeks. He continues to eat according to many of the old macrobiotic principles he had learned, but with a deeper understanding of the seasons, daily cycles, sleep, stress, exercise, and breathing. "The simplicity of the program is so elegant and its truth so self-evident that I am able to practice it without stress or strain," he later wrote to me. "No more beating myself up for failures! My afternoon cravings have completely disappeared—no more sampling handouts at the health food store, no more baked goods or chocolate cravings. I awaken more supple and flexible than I have in 10 years and I finally realize what it is like to swim downstream instead of paddling upriver all the time. I couldn't imagine eating any other way again. What a delight!"

The weight-balancing plan that I am about to lay out for you is the same plan that George took to so effortlessly. To begin with, most of the diets on the market today aim to manipulate the body to burn fat for fuel. If you are overweight and your body burns fat for energy, you will lose weight, that's for certain. By restricting fats and/or carbohydrates, many popular fad diets virtually force your body to go to its fat stores for energy. Some other diet programs use stimulants to suppress the appetite, or diuretics to flush the system. Yet unless you succeed in resetting your body's mechanism to burn fat on a steady basis, naturally and without starving it, you will simply gain back all the weight you have lost once you go off the diet (especially when you start bingeing on whatever foods were restricted by the diet).

The weight-balancing program avoids that dilemma by using different phases to help you naturally reset your body to burn fat for fuel. Just as the harvest of spring resets the body's fat-burning mechanism to prepare for the more abundant harvests of summer and fall (early winter), you will use a more stringent version of my diet to lose weight and start burning fat for fuel, then revert to a milder version on a year-round basis to maintain your ideal weight without restriction or strain. We will work up to this most demanding version of the diet gradually, through three phases.

The crucial first step, of course, is to follow the basic meal plan as often as possible on a daily basis. So let's review the elements of each meal in the 3-Season Diet. After I've explained the three-phase approach to weight loss, I'll present some tips on how to implement the plan without stress.

In nature, the best time to lose weight is during the spring, because of the natural low-fat diet it provides us. If we eat a seasonal low-fat diet during these months, the body will be forced to burn its own fat to get energy. This time of year is crucial to resetting the body's system for metabolizing fat for energy so that, come summer, when all the high-sugar fruits are harvested, the body has established a baseline of fat metabolism to maintain stable blood sugar and energy levels. The best time of year to kick off my weight-balancing program is spring. If it doesn't happen to be spring as you're reading this, you can still follow my 3-Season Plan and lose weight gradually. But if you want to be more aggressive and move the weight off a little faster, then I would suggest eating off the spring list for 1 to 3 months to force the body into fat metabolism and get the ball rolling. I would not eat against the seasonal grain for more than 3 months, however. If you do eat only from the low-fat spring diet for more than 3 months, then just as with all of the fad diets we examined earlier, the body will start to crave what it is not getting—which in this case would be the other two-thirds of nature's harvest.

Here, now, are the basics:

BREAKFAST

Start your day with one or two 8-ounce glasses of room temperature or slightly warm water. This will initiate the flushing of your kidneys and intestines first thing in the morning. If you have a small body frame, drink 1 glass; if you have a large frame, drink 2. After you exercise, shower, and dress, you are ready for breakfast. This meal should be substantial enough to get you to lunch without hunger or low energy. Depending on your activity level and your constitution, that can mean just some fruit or fruit juice. If you are unable to sustain energy on fruit alone, add small portions of toast or natural cereal, or even some eggs. Some days I don't eat anything for breakfast and cruise through to lunch without a problem. If I have a busy workload, however, I'll need a more substantial meal.

In my seminars, somebody invariably brings up the fact that on the farm, people traditionally ate a big breakfast to stoke the fires for a long workday. To which I respond that if you have a workday ahead of you that includes plowing fields, driving a tractor, pitching hay, and herding cattle, then you should eat a big farm breakfast, too, because you'll burn up all those calories before lunchtime with no problem. But if your biggest physical challenge of the morning is legging it out to the water cooler and back, you might want to hold the steak and eggs with flapjacks.

The main point of breakfast is to eat the minimum that will see you through to lunch. Once you get into the habit of eating a more generous lunch, you'll find a decreased need for both dinner and breakfast.

LUNCH

Make it the largest meal of the day. It should be a complete, large, and satisfying meal, for example: rice, chicken, vegetables, salad, soup, dessert, and herb tea. Resist the temptation to watch TV, open mail, drive your car, or talk on the phone while you eat. The thing to remember about this big lunch is that you've got to leave the table satisfied; otherwise you will crave satisfaction for the rest of the day. That's why I suggest having a dessert, even if it's only one piece of chocolate or a sweet at the end of the meal, so that you're satisfied. You should sigh with contentment as you push away from the table. Then take 5 or 10 minutes to rest.

If you feel drowsy after a big meal, lie down on your left side right after lunch for 5 or 10 minutes if you can. If that doesn't work for you, then you may want to stimulate your digestive system before the meal. Slice a gingerroot into dime-size pieces, sprinkle a little lemon juice and salt over them, and chew 2 of those before and after every meal to stimulate your digestion. You can also take gingerroot and either juice it like a carrot or use a clove press to squeeze out the juice into a little cup. You can even grate the ginger and squeeze the juice out with cheesecloth. Then add twice the amount of honey to that ginger juice, a pinch of salt, and take a tablespoon of that mixture before and after every meal.

If you still find yourself falling asleep in the afternoon, you should ask the following questions:

1. Did you eat in a rush, on the run, or in the car? If so, then make sure you slow down and eat calmly.
2. Was the food heavy or deep fried, the kind of fast food that's hard to digest? If that's the case, you've got to get better-quality food.
3. Did you jump up and go right back to work as soon as you finished eating? If so, make sure you lie down on your left side and take 5 or 10 minutes to rest and digest that meal.

There are times, however, when you need some digestive heavy artillery. I am especially found of an herb for enhancing digestion called *trikatu,* which means "three peppers" and can be found in most health food stores. Just take 1/2 teaspoon or 1 to 2 capsules before and after meals to strengthen the digestive process.

SUPPER

Remember that supper has always been a supplemental rather than a main meal. To reeducate the body to burn fat as energy instead of craving sugar and breads, this is the crucial time of the day. Most important of all, the process must be effortless. If you strain to keep from eating, then the body's emergency response will trigger cravings for more sugar (emergency fuel) and store the very fat you are trying to burn. While breakfast and lunch will remain fairly constant during your adjustment period, supper will progress from Phase One to Phase Three, but only if the process feels effortless. The goal of this program is to retrain the body to maintain its energy for a longer time by gradually decreasing the size of supper. When you can eat a large lunch and effortlessly make it through the evening without hunger, then the body will naturally and effortlessly be forced into burning its own fat for fuel. If you can maintain this diet for 2 to 4 weeks at a time, you can reset the body's ability to use fat as a natural fuel supply. Unlike other weight-loss programs that starve the body for months on end, this program pushes the body into fat metabolism each day but feeds it before the body senses any starvation emergency. Being totally satisfied with no hunger pains or cravings at night or in the afternoon is the hallmark of success.

Note: For supper in either Phase One, Two, or Three, about half an hour before your normal supper time, drink one or two 8-ounce glasses of water, even if supper is only a cup of herbal tea in Phase Three. Take 2 glasses for a larger frame and 1 or 2 for a smaller frame. This water will ensure that your hunger pains are not actually dehydration, and will help you get accurate hunger feedback from your body.

PHASE ONE

Eat soup or salad or fruit for supper. Salads work much better in the spring, fruits are better in the summer, and soup is ideal in the winter. Depending on your hunger level, of course, you can have soup and salad all year long. The kind of soup you desire may vary from season to season, but will become second nature to you very quickly. As you get comfortable with the plan, you will probably want lighter, brothy soups in the spring, almost raw soups like gazpacho in summer, and thicker, heavier soups in winter.

Phase One will be easy only if your lunch meal is large, leisurely, and satisfying. If you are not satisfied by soup, salad, or fruit for supper, then increase the size of your midday meal or eat it a little later. If you feel you need just a little something extra, however, try crumbling a few crackers in your soup, which would be a better choice for an evening carbohydrate than toast or bread. Yeasted breads will create more gas and bloating at nighttime, although many health food stores now carry delicious breads made with baking soda instead of yeast, and those would also be good in small amounts. You can always have some herb tea with raw honey in the evening to settle down your stomach.

PHASE TWO

Just as it took you 10 years to put on all that extra weight, it may take a while to get it off. Diets that promise 50-pound weight loss over a few weeks are unrealistic, and "miraculous" results tend to be undone just as miraculously. I always ask my patients, "If you can maintain 40 pounds overweight for 10 years, once we get the weight balanced why can't you maintain your ideal weight over 10 years?" If Phase one is easy then move to Phase Two: After 5:00 P.M. take only liquids, such as fruit or vegetable juice, herb tea with honey, or water.

If in the beginning you have difficulty making the transition to big lunches and light dinners, or find it impossible to make it to Phases Two and Three, take the herb *gymnema sylvester*, ½ teaspoon or 2 capsules before meals or as needed for hunger; it is available in most natural food stores. This herb is traditionally called the "sugar destroyer," because it helps the body metabolize fat as energy, stabilizes blood sugar levels, and cuts sugar cravings. Studies have shown that *gymnema* can increase the production of insulin in the beta cells of the pancreas in both Type I and Type II diabetes. I have used it successfully for years with patients who are extremely hypoglycemic and cannot tolerate sweets of any kind. In many cases people who would get dizzy and exhausted after eating sweets could now eat them in moderation. I have also seen this herb lower insulin needs in diabetic patients. It seems to reset the ability of the pancreas to make insulin and stabilize blood sugar levels. Take it for 1 to 3 months to reset the body's ability to burn fat as the primary source of energy. If evening hunger persists, give more attention to how big your lunch was and how and when you ate it; try eating your lunch later—about 3:00 or 4:00 P.M.—and drink more water (8 ounces at one time).

PHASE THREE

Only if Phases One and Two are established effortlessly do you attempt Phase Three. During this phase, you drink 3 to 6 liters of water from the end of lunch to breakfast the next morning. The word "breakfast" means exactly that, although in this case the fast you are breaking begins at the end of lunch, which may be as late as 3:00 or 4:00 P.M. Eating a big dinner at 8:00 P.M. and waking up to breakfast at 7:00 A.M. is not really breaking a fast.

To offset hunger pangs, drink 8 ounces of water (1 glass) every hour or two from the lunch meal until bedtime. Don't skip the water, because it serves an important function, helping to flush the excess fluids out of your system and filling your stomach to make you feel full. When you drink the water, you should try to drink a full 8-ounce glass at one time; don't just sip it. And if you still feel a little empty at night, have a cup of herb tea with some honey.

Phase Three prompts the body to burn fat for energy, because just about the only thing your body will have available to burn from your midday meal until breakfast *is* fat. During this daily mini-fast, the body is forced into fat metabolism without responding to it as an emergency or survival situation. During Phases Two and Three, the pancreas produces glucagon, better known as the "fasting hormone" (whereas insulin is "the feasting hormone"). Glucagon, like insulin, is a pancreatic hormone; it responds to low blood sugar levels by mobilizing stored fat as fuel. When carb availability is low, the pancreas produces glucagon to release the stored fat as energy.

When we fast from lunch to breakfast, it is not extreme or long enough to trigger acid production in the body, as high-protein diets eaten for months tend to do. But it is enough to trigger glucagon production and a powerful fat-burning response. The glucagon also ensures stable blood sugar levels that allow an individual to have a consistent energy level rather than the peak-and-valley variety associated with excessive carbohydrate intake. This may take a few weeks to develop, which is why I recommend a three-phase program so you can gracefully reeducate your body to burn fat as fuel and make energy last without putting any strain on the body.

If you can stay with Phase Three for 3 to 4 weeks, you'll watch the weight fall off. I lost 20 pounds in 4 weeks following this regimen. George, as we saw, lost 10 pounds in 2 weeks, and other patients reported similar weight losses. But if you find it too difficult to stay on Phase Three for a week, try it for 1 day, and the next day go back to Phase One. The day after that, if you're not ready to return to Phase Three, do Phase Two, then go back to Phase One. Even if you just alternate between the three phases, you'll still be on an accelerated weight-loss, fat-burning program. It may take you a little longer to lose the weight, but you will. You may find that, depending on what kind of day you have had, you will be more inclined to do Phase One, Two, or Three. If you had a hectic day and couldn't get a satisfactory lunch, do Phase One that evening. If all went well and lunch was large and relaxed, then do Phase Two or Three. The idea is to gracefully retain the body to be able to make energy for the long haul. Instead of needing food every two hours, you are establishing slow-burning fat cells as a prime energy source. As soon as this begins to happen, you will depend on carbs less and less for your physical and mental energy.

Often the weight will fall off in ten to fifteen pound stages with each stage lasting about a month. If you notice your weight loss progress slowing down after a month of Phase Two or Three, then go back to Phase One for four to six days. This will send a message to your body that this process is not a fat-storing emergency. Then if more weight loss is desired, do Phase Three for another month.

The best news is that once you have lost your target weight, you simply revert to a relaxed Phase One and that becomes your year-round eating regimen. After you have lost the weight, it is not essential that you eat only soup, salad, or fruit for supper, although that may well be all you desire. At that stage you can be a little more flexible, understanding that supper is a small, supplemental meal, and avoiding large helpings of meat, breads, and pasta.

If you do eat a heavy dinner and know you are going to feel heavy in the morning, then take some digestive aids before and after that big evening meal. This way you'll have a better chance of digesting it with a minimum of upset. Try the ginger recipes mentioned above, or the herb *trikatu* before and after that meal. This is the best way to mitigate an off-the-plan pizza and ice cream bash at midnight!

Of course, you can enjoy a big dinner on occasion, as long as you understand that it is not the norm. On those days, just eat a light lunch, relax, and feel good about yourself. What you do every day is what will make a difference in your life, not what you do once in a while. Once you start this process of eating large meals at midday and lighter dinners at night, you will find that your energy becomes more stable, your digestion is stronger, and you will have much more resiliency to go out and break the rules without suffering an extreme case of the blahs the morning after. But remember that if every day of your life you go against the grain, then your comfort zone with food will shrink as you get older.

When Alice came to see me a few years ago, she was about 60 pounds overweight, chronically fatigued, with high blood pressure and extreme environmental sensitivity—meaning that she could barely leave her house. She suffered from multiple allergies and could not take any medications because of the extreme side effects she suffered, which left her blood pressure uncontrolled. Because of her chronic fatigue symptoms, Alice had found it difficult to hold down a job for almost 2 years. She came to see me because her strong reactions to any and all medications and even herbs left both allopathic and complementary practitioners unable to help her.

Alice was trying to lose weight because, among other reasons, her doctors had told her that her overweight was responsible for her high blood pressure. To lower her caloric intake, she was advised to eat a salad and cottage cheese for lunch, but this regimen left her craving coffee, Coke, and chocolate all afternoon. Because these light lunches were not satisfying her energy needs, she was resorting to emergency fuel in the form of sugar and caffeine. I began by explaining the logic of the 3-Season Diet and why her typically big dinners were so hard for her to digest. I urged her to eat her larger meal in the middle of the day and have just soup and salad for dinner. I told her to relax during this large midday meal and take 5 minutes to rest afterward, followed by a short walk if possible. I also taught her the weight-loss techniques associated with breathing that I will discuss in the following chapters, and I told her to come back and see me in 2 weeks.

Because Alice's environmental sensitivity precluded her using supplements of any sort, I focused on how and when she ate her meals and how she breathed. Two weeks later she had a checkup with her local physician, and to his surprise, her blood pressure had gone down and she was 10 pounds lighter. Alice reported that she also felt considerably more energy, so we were well on our way. I was soon able to give her some gentle herbs, including *gymnema sylvester* to stabilize her blood sugar and improve her energy, and for once she had no adverse reaction to these supplements. Within 3 months, Alice had lost 25 pounds, her blood pressure was normal, her energy was back, and she was able to nail down a prestigious position. A year later she had lost 50 pounds and today, a few years later, she is eating effortlessly with the seasons.

THE CHOLESTEROL BLUES

One of the side effects of weight gain is high cholesterol. As I have mentioned, many cholesterol-lowering diets and drugs work for some of the people some of the time. Yet a large number of people achieve only moderate levels of success from these diets or drugs. Remember that when the body craves sugar, bread, coffee, or cola, it is forcing itself to raise insulin levels. Consistently high insulin levels, often induced by constant mental, emotional, or physical stressors, will cause the body to store fat and raise cholesterol levels. Cholesterol is a sterol that is a precursor to cortisol and other degenerative, stress-fighting hormones. In an emergency the body says, "Hold the fat! Make me some more cholesterol to replace the steroid hormones I'm using in this emergency!" This scenario has become all too common in America for many of the reasons we have already outlined.

One herb has been shown to lower cholesterol levels as well as commercial Western drugs. It has no side effects—although it does offer a number of side *benefits* for healing skin irritations, arthritis, and other conditions. The herb is called *comminphora mukul,* or more commonly, *guggul.* It will lower cholesterol to normal levels, yet studies have shown that if taken continually it does not bring cholesterol levels below normal. *Guggul* seems to act by restoring homeostasis, or balance, to the entire body rather than only addressing symptoms. The standard dose for this herb is 300 mg, three times a day for 3 months, followed by a reevaluation of your cholesterol levels. I have seen many cholesterol ratings in the high 200s and low 300s drop into the low 200s and 180s after 3 months of using *guggul.* It is also known to detoxify fat cells, so it serves several valuable functions at once, and can be an important part of a weight-balancing program.

INSULIN RESISTANCE

Insulin, produced by the pancreas in response to the release of glucose in the bloodstream, carries the glucose to the body's tissues either for use as energy or to be converted to fat for storage. When insulin levels are kept high over an extended period of time because of stress or an extended high-carb diet (the carbs break down ultimately to sugar), a condition called insulin resistance may result. While under stress, the adrenal glands produce cortisol and the body dumps all available glycogen or sugar into the blood. Insulin levels rise to get the blood into the cells. If the insulin levels stay high for too long, the cells cannot use all the sugar the stress is trying to force into the cell with high insulin levels. The cell will eventually block the insulin from driving any more sugar into it.

The body soon starts to have difficulty digesting carbs at all—a situation called "insulin resistance." The pancreas has to keep making more insulin to get the sugar into the cells for energy. With this cellular insulin resistance, the body is getting a very strong message to store fat, make cholesterol, and crave more carbs. Does that sound familiar?

In this case, my three-phase program may need a boost, since over time the pancreas will begin to fatigue and not be able to produce enough insulin. The herb *gymnema* mentioned above would be perfect to enhance the beta cells in the pancreas to make insulin more efficiently. If the pancreas fails to make the insulin, the blood sugars rise uncontrollably and you become diabetic, needing insulin support. Prior to this, diet and lifestyle stress will also keep insulin unnaturally high. In time the cells become insulin-resistant and the body resists taking the glycogen into the cells. To counteract this I recommend another natural medicine called *shilijit*, or bitumen. This medicine has been shown to take the blood sugar into the cells and lower insulin resistance, and for this reason it has traditionally been used for diabetes, increasing energy, and fighting obesity. Take 1 or 2 capsules of *shilijit* after meals and 1 or 2 *gymnema* before meals. When combined, *gymnema* and *shilijit* can have a powerful impact on insulin-resistant weight problems. Once those are solved, the three-phase program should work like a charm.

THE DEPRESSION–WEIGHT LOSS CONNECTION

As I described in the story of my patient named Jason (see page 4), depression and weight gain can often be linked to low serotonin levels in the brain. When serotonin levels are low, the brain craves carbohydrates, which increase the absorption of the neurotransmitter tryptophan into the brain. Tryptophan stimulates the production of serotonin, generating a sense of well-being.

Many of today's most popular antidepressants, such as Prozac and Zoloft, work by increasing serotonin levels. When we experience either mental, emotional, or physical stress, cortisol levels rise and the body craves carbs. Insulin levels also rise, flooding the body with blood sugar and the brain with tryptophan, which in turn stimulates the production of more mood-enhancing serotonin. The problem with this scenario is that by the time the brain gets its serotonin levels high enough to stabilize mood, the body has already craved and binged on an excess of fat-storing carbohydrates. This is the body chemistry behind the term "emotional eating"–the reflex attempt to counteract depressed moods and serotonin starvation with uncontrollable bingeing on carbs.

For the most part, we can eliminate cravings with the 3-Season Diet and the weight-balancing program described in this chapter. In some cases, however, there is a problem with the brain chemistry, and serotonin levels stay dangerously low. For certain body types this can perpetuate the carbohydrate bingeing and uncontrollable weight gain. In my practice I sometimes have to supplement the weight-balancing program with an herb that stabilizes serotonin levels naturally. In the brain there is an enzyme that destroys serotonin called monoamine oxidase, or MAO. Without adequate amounts of serotonin, you can experience headaches, depression, sleeplessness, decreased short-term memory, and the above-mentioned weight gain and cravings. Certain natural medicines act as MAO inhibitors, meaning that they block MAO from destroying the serotonin. One of these herbs has become well known as a natural antidepressant, but few people realize its value in controlling weight and cravings. *Hypericum perforatum,* better known as Saint-John's-wort, is an MAO inhibitor that naturally raises serotonin levels so that the body doesn't crave carbs and doesn't need to wait so long to get stable. Saint-John's-wort can act as a preventative to keep the brain chemistry stable while the 3-Season Diet and weight-balancing program reset the fat-burning and sugar-stabilizing processes of the body. Take Saint-John's-wort 30 to 40 minutes before a meal or as needed for cravings. About 30 to 40 drops of an extract three or four times a day should help.

Needless to say, there is no good in using any of the herbal recommendations for symptomatic relief without changing the way you live. These herbs can help the body restore normal brain and blood sugar chemistries, but keep in mind that living against the grain was what pushed the chemistry out of balance in the first place. These herbs are for short-term use with the goal of achieving balanced weight and stable moods without creating a dependency on anything—even a natural herb.

CONSTIPATED?

Recently a patient I hadn't seen in 5 or 6 years returned for a visit. At first I didn't recognize her, until she told me that she had lost 45 pounds. When I asked her how she did it, she reminded me that I had prescribed an herb for her to take after meals to stimulate elimination, because she had a history of slow digestion and constipation. (If you are not eliminating well, you will not be able to lose weight effectively.) Since she had been taking 2 capsules of this herb after every meal, her digestion and lifelong constipation had normalized, and she had gradually begun to lose weight. It took her 2 or 3 years to lose the whole 45 pounds, but it happened so easily for her that she never felt she was straining or suffering.

The herb I had given her is called *triphala,* a commonly available combination of three bitter and astringent fruits. As we get more constipated over time, the gut often becomes increasingly distended and gradually loses its ability to contract and squeeze out waste. So many people are addicted to strong fibers like psyllium because they swell up in the intestines and push against the distended colon to make it contract. But fiber also pulls a lot of the water out of the gut and can dry it over time, leaving it expanded and nonresponsive to the fiber. Because *triphala* is not a laxative, it tonifies the bowel and makes it contract naturally, while pulling the mucus out of the intestines and repairing damage to intestinal tissue with powerful antioxidant agents.

MENOPAUSE AND WEIGHT GAIN

Many women complain of weight gain after menopause or after taking hormone replacement therapy. Estrogens naturally tell the body to hold on to fat, which is why ranchers feed their cows estrogens to beef them up for slaughter. Therefore estrogen replacement can present some complications when you are trying to lose weight. Naturally derived estrogens and progesterones available on the market today can help you in this regard. I also recommend certain herbs that act as hormonal precursors, such as asparagus root, or *shatavari*, and wild yam extract (Dioscorea). In addition, an herb called chaste tree berry *(Vitex agnus)* helps the pituitary to release stimulating hormones that tell the body to make estrogens and progesterones.

PORTIONS

Some years ago I took a vacation on St. Barts, a Caribbean island in the French West Indies. It was my first experience with French food—and French prices. We ordered lunch by the pool, and when my salad and sandwich came, I couldn't believe my eyes. The salad consisted of a few pieces of lettuce, a few carrots, maybe a piece of celery, and some fancy garnishes, and the sandwich was about one-quarter the size of what I would usually eat in the States. There wasn't enough food to feed a mouse, I thought, yet with just a glass of lemonade the bill came to $35! I was in shock. It took me a few days to get accustomed to the French style of eating, but once I did I came to realize that although the portions were small, a surprising amount of preparation went into the food. I came to enjoy that tiny salad, for instance, with its marinated carrots, velvety lettuce, and subtle but extremely tasty dressing laced with herbs I couldn't quite identify. I realized that if I slowed down enough to savor the food instead of inhaling it in my usual fashion, I probably would not need to eat as much as I thought.

The portions we have become accustomed to here in America are exceptional when compared to the rest of the world. Because of our extraordinary abundance and low food prices, most of the time we simply overeat by force of habit. Most of us have never slowed down long enough to enjoy the process of eating the way people do in other cultures. Back in the 1980s, French-inspired nouvelle cuisine was introduced in America—smaller portions of more elegantly prepared and often exotically flavored foods meant to be savored for their surprising combinations of different ingredients and tastes. Yet much of the criticism this trend faced came from people who complained, just as I did on St. Barts, that it was an excuse to charge too much for portions that were too small. As if taste didn't matter at all!

And so my advice to anyone who wants to lose weight is to begin by experimenting with eating only until you are full. Be sure that you are relaxed and not rushed when you eat. We can learn from our kids in this regard: They eat until they are full; then they stop and leave the table. We sometimes tell them to eat everything on their plate, but they know better. (Their food selection could be more informed, of course, but that may come in time.) If you do not finish the food on your own plate, it's all right. Soon you will be accustomed to smaller portions and will take only what you need—enjoying it all the more with longer-lasting energy.

During the midday meal, as I have said, I want you to eat well but leisurely. The more relaxed you are, the more food you can comfortably digest. If you inhale a large meal without paying conscious attention, you will surely be nodding off at your desk by 3:00 P.M. But as you become more aware of your eating habits in terms of when you eat, how you eat, and what you eat, you will naturally derive more nutrition from less food. Along the way you will become more particular about the food you choose. Chances are that a quick bite of a fast-food burger and fries just won't be all that appealing anymore. To trade in a nice, relaxing meal of well-prepared food for a Big Mac will sound like a silly proposition.

When I first embarked on my own weight-balancing program, I jumped directly to Phase Three and ate a huge lunch including three veggie burgers, soup, salad, and a couple of brownies. I wanted to make sure I would not starve, since I was planning to have only water for supper. At 8:00 P.M. I was still stuffed and couldn't think about eating more food. Even with such an excessive lunch portion, I continued to lose weight. Within a week or so, however, I realized that I wasn't going to starve or suffer hunger pains at night if I didn't eat such huge portions. Once my body (and mind) became convinced that it could handle it effortlessly, I became quite satisfied with smaller portions.

In India they say that if you eat one meal a day you're a *yogi;* two meals a day, you're a *rhogi*—one who does not have strong willpower; and three meals a day, you're a *bhogi*—one who is attached to every worldly thing. Only in America do we feel entitled to eat three substantial meals a day. Our stomachs have been distended to the point where we eat far beyond our hunger levels. In many cases we are eating emotionally, and part of the reason we eat emotionally is that we've been feeling undernourished all afternoon. We didn't eat sufficiently at the one time of day when the body could handle a large meal, so we binge on dinner. You won't believe the feeling of relief once you discover that a single large meal, eaten at the optimal time of day, with a supplemental breakfast and dinner, is all you really need to be both comfortable and healthy.

THE OXYGEN MASK PRINCIPLE

I promised earlier that I would offer some suggestions for incorporating the big lunch into a culture and a way of life that seems to militate against it. Based on my own experience and that of the thousands of patients whom I've treated, I have developed a number of strategies that succeed remarkably well in a variety of family and work situations. With five young kids, three of whom are now in school, it has been a challenge to follow my own program, believe me! If you have kids, the secret to making the big lunch concept work is what I call "The Oxygen Mask Principle." Whenever I take an airplane and the fight attendants begin their rap about exit doors and flotation cushions, I generally zone out while trying to look attentive, and reach for a magazine or a good book. But one line has always caught my attention—the one about what to do when there's a change in cabin pressure and those little yellow masks drop out of the ceiling. The attendants tell you that if you have small children, *make sure to put on your own oxygen mask first, then take care of your kids.* This goes against the instincts of most parents to protect kids first, but the logic is inescapable. If you fumble around trying to get that mask on a cranky, scared 3-year-old when your own blood pressure and respiration rate are rising, you may well black out before you accomplish your task, and you will both perish.

I try to follow the same principle when it comes to eating. Whether at home or in a restaurant, my wife, Ginger, and I sit down in the middle of the day and have a meal together in a relaxed setting. Come dinnertime, we're already feeling nourished, our blood sugar is under control, and we can munch on a salad or sip a bowl of soup while focusing more intently on the kids. We don't feel frazzled or deprived, and the kids like getting our full attention. But if all you've had is a cottage cheese and tuna fish kind of lunch and the kids come home from school after having eaten little or none of their cafeteria lunch, around four o'clock you've got a situation not unlike that scene on the airplane where everybody is gasping for breath.

Besides, if you have some decent food waiting for the kids when they get home, they're usually so ravenous, they'll eat anything—yes, folks, even sautéed veggies, rice, beans, and tofu! The trick is to get 'em when they're desperate. The hot lunches many schools serve are, in most of the kids' minds, not so hot. Between the warmed-over pizza, "rubber" hot dogs, and overcooked pasta, they'd rather grab a dessert and rush out to the schoolyard to play with their friends. You don't necessarily have to stay home and cook big meals for your kids to see that they get decent nutrition, either. Most health food stores and many supermarkets now carry a variety of dehydrated vegetable and noodle soups without additives that just need boiling water to turn into a fairly substantial meal that most teenagers can make for themselves. You can have those soups waiting for the kids along with good breads and maybe some sandwich material. It doesn't have to be a four-course meal with all the trimmings, but it should be more substantial than a bowl of commercial cereal with extra sugar.

Although hot lunches in the school cafeteria are not a big hit with most kids, the origin of the concept lies in the agricultural society we have so recently left. In a previous era, it was mainly the children of the upper classes who got educated; the kids of agricultural laborers worked in the fields with them or helped with chores. As society evolved to the point where farm children could be sent to public schools, the farmers wanted to be sure that their kids would be fed in the same way they would be at home—and the hot-meal program for schoolkids was born. The hot-lunch program that survives in many of today's schools is one of the last remnants of a time when we all ate big lunches and light suppers. As the West became fully industrialized, most countries kept their eating habits intact; in the United States, unfortunately, we changed the rules and soon became the fattest nation in the world. And not only are our children becoming obese at a world-leading pace, they are developing related health problems as well.

Not long ago an elementary school child was brought to me suffering from attention deficit disorder and severe blood sugar problems. When I interviewed him, I discovered that his two best friends had their lunch period just before his. He would wolf down his food as fast as possible, or skip lunch altogether, so he could race out to play with his friends for the last ten minutes of their recess. As I've already pointed out, your brain wants 80 percent of your blood sugar during the afternoon hours, and this kid was quite literally running on empty. With no real food to fuel his nervous system in the afternoon, his classroom attention was severely diminished. (For much the same reason, many offices pass around the chocolates in the afternoon; the employees' starving brains are demanding emergency fuel in the form of the four c's—cola, coffee, chocolate, or chips.)

When he came home from school, this boy would have a typical American kid's snack: either cereal with milk and plenty of sugar, cupcakes, doughnuts, or some other sugar-based food. After a couple of years of eating like that, his blood sugar was off the charts. When I saw him, he was hyperactive and complaining of dizziness; he had been put on a whole litany of drugs, including ritalin, but none of the doctors who prescribed those drugs had ever thought to ask the kid about his diet or what he ate for lunch. When a young child's brain doesn't have enough of the right food, the kid will either become spaced out or hyperactive from the release of stress-fighting hormones, which tend to be highly stimulating. To make matters even worse, this boy was drinking a lot of diet sodas laced with a popular aspartame-based artificial sweetener (NutraSweet) that, because of its stimulating properties, has been clinically linked anecdotally with ADD.

What this poor kid was experiencing has been happening on a slightly smaller scale to large numbers of schoolkids across America. They come home after eating very little lunch, have a quick, sugar-based snack, then go outside and run around for a couple of hours, or play video games that get them completely wired. By the time their parents tell them to settle down and start their homework, they have lost any ability to concentrate. And when it's time for supper, parents struggle to get them to eat a green vegetable when all the kids want is another glass of soda. When their blood sugar has hit bottom and the kids are craving more sugar, vegetables are the last thing on their mind. Then it's another battle to get the kids to go to sleep early when they're still wired.

Often my patients will say, "I can't go out and have a big lunch, because when I come home, my family still wants to eat a big dinner together." The fallacy in that statement is contained in the word "together." When I was in India, I noticed something startling the first few times I was invited to someone's home for dinner or lunch: The mother would serve everybody but never sit down to eat herself. Occasionally she would sit at the edge of the table for a few moments and join in the conversation, but then would race back into the kitchen. Even in the most conservative households in America, I had never seen anything like this. I began to feel very uncomfortable during these meals, and ascribed it to the generally poor treatment of women in India.

Then after one of these meals I walked through the kitchen to go to the backyard and saw the woman of the house sitting all by herself in a quiet setting, peacefully eating her meal. As I observed her tranquil demeanor, I wondered if she didn't prefer eating like this to to grabbing quick bites in between all the courses that make up a typical middle-class Indian meal. Yet that's the way most American parents eat—grabbing a bite, jumping up to get some more food for the kids, sitting down and grabbing another bite, cleaning up the mess that the toddlers make, and never relaxing for a minute. All things considered, you're better off taking care of your own needs first and being better prepared to give your kids the nutrition they need.

THE 51 PERCENT RULE

Keep in mind that my big lunch system will work with many variations. If you can't do it every day of the work week, perhaps you can try it two days a week; then on the weekends you can make a big lunch at home on Saturday and take your family out to brunch on Sunday. If you eat your main meal at midday just four days a week, you're still doing it the majority of the time. And you're accomplishing one of the goals of the 3-Season Diet, which is to reset your metabolism to burn fat. So even if you're not eating perfectly every day, you *are* burning fat for fuel on some level. This is what I call The 51 Percent Rule. If you are doing this program 51 percent of the time, then for the majority of your life you are going downstream, not against the current.

When I first started developing this diet for myself, I didn't have a life that allowed me to follow it every single day. It took many years for me to structure my life and my practice so that I could control how and when I ate. In my first practice, I was working with other doctors and I couldn't just say that I wanted to come to work an hour earlier and take two hours for lunch, because it wasn't my practice. Now I have my own situation and I can call my own shots, and I've been able to adjust my life to my dietary principles. After 15 years of perfecting this diet, I'm still getting better at it, and still enjoying the process of getting better at it. I'll be doing this for the rest of my life, but I understand that in the beginning the big lunch may not be the easiest thing in the world to implement.

Patients of mine who are elementary and high school teachers often complain that they don't have enough time to stop and have a large meal in the middle of the day, because they have to attend meetings or be on cafeteria patrol during their lunch hour. Many of them get out of school between 2:30 and 4:00 P.M., however, and have the option of going home and having their big meal at that time. It may not be ideal, but it's still a lot better than dinner at 8:00 P.M. They often typically go out for a walk or a workout or run errands right after school, and then come home and have a big dinner after sunset. Just switching those two activities–going home and eating first, then exercising at 6:00 P.M.–can make a huge difference in terms of how much time you give your body to digest your food. If you run on empty all day long and then fuel up when you get home, you shouldn't be surprised if you feel exhausted.

If you work at home, as more and more people are doing these days, you can easily find ways to arrange your schedule around a big midday meal. You'll discover that the increased productivity more than makes up for any inconvenience; at 2:00 P.M., when your brain wants 80 percent of your blood sugar for the day, you'll have a full tank of gas. You won't be craving emergency fuel and triggering degenerative hormone and free-radical production, and you will no longer answer yes to those two big questions: Do you feel exhausted at the end of your day? and Do you crave sweets, chips, soda, or coffee in the afternoon?

But what if you work in an office in the city? You can't take 2 hours off and you can't go home for lunch, so what do you do? A friend of mine whom I'll call Dave supplied the answer to that question after he and his wife spent a week during the summer vacationing on Nantucket Island, off the coast of Massachusetts. Nantucket is a lovely spot no more than 11 miles wide, and you don't need a car to get around; you just take the ferry and rent bicycles on the island. The first two nights there, Dave and his wife, Linda, ate big dinners at a couple of Nantucket's many fine restaurants. These luxurious dinners left them feeling bloated the next day, so they ate very little breakfast and experienced low energy when they went out to ride their bikes. The dinner scenario was creating other problems, too. Because the best restaurants are so busy during the summer tourist season, it was difficult to get reservations, so Dave and Linda had to shape their entire evening around whatever time slot was available for dinner.

On the third day of their vacation, they were biking through town at midday when they noticed that one of the best restaurants on the island, which had been packed the night before, was open and almost completely empty. The lunch menu in the window showed prices that were considerably less than those for dinner. They locked their bikes, strolled in without a reservation, and ordered a sumptuous lunch, which they took their time eating. The waitress was only too happy to have customers to serve, and there was no pressure to hurry and make room for the next guests; she provided attentive service and chatted amiably. They stayed long after they had finished eating and digested their food.

After a short stroll, Dave and his wife resumed their biking and had plenty of energy the rest of the day. They realized, as they were returning to their hotel room later that evening, that they had no desire for dinner, so they just stopped off for a bowl of soup and enjoyed a restful night's sleep. Dave and Linda were hungry the next morning and enjoyed the hotel's complimentary continental breakfast of cereal and fruit. Then they checked the restaurant listings and discovered to their delight that all the places where they had been struggling to get dinner reservations also served lunch. In each case they ate the same wonderful food at lower prices, never needed a reservation, and weren't rushed through their meals. When they ordered wine with lunch at one Italian restaurant, the owner brought Dave down to the wine cellar and let hm pick out his own bottle.

The result of their new eating schedule was that they had energy to burn. On lovely evenings they would stroll to one of the waterfront restaurants and have a bowl of soup or a plate of oysters, not needing anything more than that. When they returned home after the week was over, Dave and Linda were pleased to discover that they had not gained any weight, as they had on their last vacation, and were in better shape from all their walking and bicycling. They began trying as often as possible to eat big lunches at home, and very light dinners. Their energy levels improved and over time they actually lost weight. But the best part came when Linda went back to work in the city. She discovered plenty of good restaurants where meals at lunchtime are almost half the price for the same food. Even better, she tried out some of the restaurants offering buffet lunches–all you can eat for as little as $5.00 or $6.00! Chinese, Mexican, Japanese, Indian, Thai, and other restaurants featuring ethnic cuisine all had attractive lunch specials or buffets. Even with just an hour for lunch, she could walk in, fill up her plate with anything from chicken and broccoli in garlic sauce to tandoori salmon and spinach, sit down, eat it in a relaxed way, and take 10 minutes to digest it. An hour later she would be back at work fueled up and ready for a long afternoon at her desk.

In Boulder, Colorado, where I live, they have a service that will deliver a meal from any one of more than fifty restaurants for a $2.00 charge, something other cities are beginning to offer. So even if you can't leave work, you can still have good food delivered at reasonable prices. When the food comes, just turn off your computer and go to the dining area, or close your office door, and take a good half hour to eat in a comfortable way. By law in most states, your employer has to allow you at least a half hour for lunch. I even tell my patients to inform the boss that their doctor said it's urgent that because of their blood sugar levels, they take a full half hour and have a big main meal. Nobody has ever reported back that their boss refused to allow it. Many corporations are already ahead of me on that one, anyway. They have realized that productivity levels are so dramatically reduced in the afternoon that they are insisting their people leave the building for an hour during lunchtime.

Even if your employer isn't so enlightened, you still have options. Many of my patients cook big soups the night before and put them in thermoses to take to work. Most offices have microwaves and refrigerators, but instead of eating low-nutrition frozen dinners, you can use the microwave to heat up big plates of cooked veggies or roast chicken and rice from home. The most important thing is to create enough time for yourself to eat a big meal, even if half an hour is all you can get right now. This is not to say that I am a fan of microwaves or frozen foods, but you have to pick your battles. It is better to eat at the right time of day and in a relaxed way by having your food prepared earlier and heated up than to eat fast-food junk in a rush.

Let's say you work as a nurse or firefighter, someone who may be called to an emergency in the middle of the day, and won't have an hour to sit down until 3:00 P.M. even if your lunch break is supposed to be at 1:00 P.M. When 3:00 P.M. comes around, many people will just go downstairs and grab a sandwich and start eating it on the way back up the elevator. Or they think, "It's already three. I'll just have a doughnut and a cup of coffee to hold me until dinner tonight." By the time they get home they're not only ravenous, they're also a little light headed, exhausted from having worked on an empty stomach, wired from caffeine, and will stuff themselves for the sheer emotional satisfaction of a filling meal, not realizing that they won't be able to digest it fully.

Studies have shown that working the late shift affects most people's health adversely, and many cities now require alternating shifts for employees such as police and firefighters. But if you have to work late at night, you can still go home, get to bed, wake up at around 1:00 or 2:00 P.M., and have your big meal then. Even though you're not totally on the cycle, you'll be giving your body sufficient time to digest that big meal, and you won't be tempted to eat so many snack foods at work. One patient of mine is a baker whose workday is over by noon. He can go home and have a big meal before 2:00 P.M., rest awhile, exercise, run errands, and still get to bed early enough to be up at 11:00 A.M. the next day.

I mentioned how Dave and Linda transformed their vacation by eating a big lunch. With five kids, my wife and I have had to develop some survival strategies of our own while on vacation. After a morning swim, we often hit the breakfast buffet about 11:00 A.M., just before it closes. By then the crowd has usually gone and we have the whole buffet to ourselves. This one main meal in early midday usually lasts us until supper time. Keep in mind that kids have to eat three square meals a day, however; we always feed them based on their hunger levels. Kids generally know when to eat and how much to eat—even if their choice of *what* to eat has been warped by modern culture and children's advertising.

People from cultures around the world are often appalled when they see Americans eating their meals in front of the computer or while they're in the middle of their work. Throughout the world, eating has traditionally been a sacred act and a time to thank God, and requires at the very least that we be calm and reflective so we can absorb the nutrition that nature is giving us. I believe that this was also one of the purposes of saying grace: not only to thank the Creator for the gift of food but also to admire that gift, to slow the mind and increase our awareness that this food is what we will become! Eating food in traditional cultures is a communication between the intelligence of nature expressed as the food and our own inner intelligence, sometimes referred to as our consciousness. When I returned from my first trip to India, I spent eight years codirecting Deepak Chopra's health center in Massachusetts. At that time we were attracting a number of cancer patients, many of whom had been given 6 months to a year to live by their doctors. After working with these terminal patients, I would often hear comments such as the following testimonial from one of our many visitors:

"Do you know the most important thing I learned during my week here? I learned how to eat! I used to eat as if I were fueling up my car with gas—just fill up as fast as I could and get back on the road. I now realize that how I eat is extremely important. I can't just gobble my food and race back to work, expecting to digest that food and stay healthy. Now I see that eating is sacred, as it is in every traditional culture we have studied."

Of all the things these patients could have said about their week of rejuvenation, the fact that so many of them commented on their atrocious eating habits made a strong impression on me. Eating became the primary activity that they resolved to change after leaving our center to help prolong their lives or beat cancer. A dozen years later, some of these "terminal" patients are still around to testify to the value of conscious eating.

I realize that you still may have days when your schedule is so packed that work doesn't allow you time for a leisurely lunch during which you can relax, thank God, and savor your food. So just remember the 51 Percent Principle, and eat that big lunch as often as you can. Once your body gets a taste of what life is like when swimming with the current, you will find that your desire to eat this way grows naturally. Soon, instead of 51 percent of the time, you will be doing it 80 or 90 percent because you love the way you feel.

CHAPTER 10

Breathing for Life

O NE OF THE BODY'S major nervous systems is called the
autonomic, or involuntary, nervous system, which can automatically push the body into either a fight-or-flight response
or a calming, repairing, rejuvenating response. Those two responses are
controlled by what is known as the sympathetic nervous system and the
parasympathetic nervous system, respectively. Most of us live in a way
that triggers the sympathetic nervous system on an almost continuous
basis, with the result that we are constantly perceiving life as an emergency. The goal of my weight-balancing program is to allow the sympathetic and parasympathetic nervous systems to coexist as more equal
partners. The autonomic nervous system was named according to the
belief that we had no conscious control over its function. Research has
shown, however, that this automatic nervous system *can* be controlled
by the way you breathe.

In the course of a single day, we take approximately 28,000 breaths.
Can you think of any other action that you have control over and that
you will do 28,000 times a day? Your heart may beat more often than
that, but unless you practice advanced forms of yoga, it's not something
you can consciously control. You do, however, have quite a bit of control over the way you breathe, and how you breathe can very directly
affect how you feel physically, mentally, and emotionally. Most of us
walk around breathing like rabbits, taking short, shallow breaths all day
long—a little air in, a little air out. Because the rib cage possesses what's

called elastic recoil, it is squeezing down on your heart and lungs all day in an effort to get the air out—which is a good thing. But if you add a little stress to that normal recoil, the ribs can begin to feel more and more like a cage that's growing tighter and tighter.

What's worse, those shallow, rapid breaths I mentioned activate the sympathetic stress receptors that predominate in the upper lobes of the lungs. These stress receptors are designed to trigger responses that are beneficial *during emergencies.* Sympathetic activity increases heart rate, constricts blood vessels to make circulation more efficient in an emergency, and increases blood pressure. At the same time, digestion slows down, stress-fighting hormones are released, damaging free radicals are produced, insulin and cholesterol levels increase, and fat is not only stored but blocked from being utilized for fuel. As we have seen, such effects are not good for our longevity if they occur repeatedly. And just as burning sugar for energy on a regular basis is ultimately deleterious to our health, it is debilitating to activate those stress receptors in the upper lobes on a regular basis.

But that is precisely what happens when you exercise in the conventional manner, huffing and puffing into the upper chest while you run, bike, or lift weights. When you realize that you can actually gain weight for your efforts, it's not surprising that 80 percent of Americans do not exercise on a regular basis.

How you breathe will determine whether your body responds to exercise as a fat-storing emergency or a fat-burning experience. If you look at Figure 1, you will see that when the intensity of exercise goes up, the body burns more carbs and less fat. When the intensity declines, the body burns more fat and fewer carbs. This chart makes clear that, contrary to popular belief, the harder you push when you exercise the *less* fat you will burn. To make matters worse, because you burn more carbs, you will crave them after the workout.

When you follow my instructions and learn how to breathe into the lower lobes of the lungs, where the calming receptors are, you will be telling your body that exercise is not an emergency. That means it can burn nonemergency fuel, which is fat. When we teach your body how to handle higher and higher levels of stress without responding to the exertion as an emergency, your body will learn how to burn more and more fat as a natural source of fuel rather than sugar. Couple this to the eating program that we discussed in Part I of this book, and now you have a way to multiply the amount of fat burning your body will do on a regular basis.

You have three choices for breathing techniques during vigorous exercise: chest and clavicular breathing; diaphragmatic breathing; and what I call "whole lung" breathing. The last is neither belly breathing nor diaphragmatic breathing but rather a method in which all the lobes of the lungs work together. This is the most efficient means of respiration, and the most beneficial; sadly, it is the least common in our society. With their underdeveloped chests, infants and young children are restricted from using the entire chest to breathe. Most commonly the lower lobes of the lungs–which have a powerful calming influence that is remarkably similar to the "runner's high" many athletes experience during exercise–become blocked owing to a natural "elastic recoil" or squeezing on the rib cage, and kids are forced to breathe like rabbits, using only the upper lobes, where the stress receptors are located.

What I call chest and clavicular breathing is performed largely by

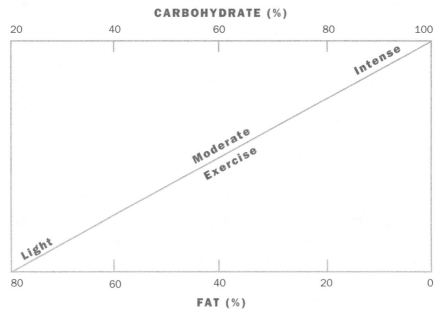

Figure 1. Energy utilization during exercise. Note. From Sharkey (1984).

expanding and lifting the rib cage via the intercostal muscles. When we are desperate for air, we even raise our clavicles, or collarbones, to lengthen the chest cavity. This happens not only during physical exertion but often under emotional stress as well. When you heave a sigh of despair, you are desperate for more oxygen (as you are to a lesser extent when you yawn). Ironically, this action is more taxing than diaphragmatic breathing and requires more work and a higher heart rate. Chest breathing fills the middle and upper portions of the lungs but doesn't efficiently engage the blood-rich lower lobes. This procedure allows you to get large quantities of air in and out of the upper and middle lobes, but the more ample blood supply needed for a quality exchange, especially during oxygen-demanding exercise, is in the lower lobes. To get enough oxygen through chest breathing, both breath and heart rates must be faster.

What is valuable about "whole lung" breathing is that, if done correctly, it pulls air into the lower lungs first as we inhale by contracting the diaphragm, a flat, parachute-shaped muscle at the base of the lungs. The blood supply to the lower lobes is dependent on gravity, so that while we are upright, far more blood is available for oxygen exchange in the lower parts of the lungs. As the diaphragm contracts and flattens out on inhalation, the lower rib cage expands and the abdomen feels protruded. During exhalation, the natural elastic recoil of the lungs and tension on their inner surface will retract the lungs, create the dome shape of the relaxed diaphragm, and expel carbon dioxide (CO_2) and other gases. To expel the CO_2 completely from the lower lobes, the abdominal muscles have to engage and squeeze out the residual air.

You can try this right now. As you exhale normally, you'll see that to squeeze the last bit of air out of your lungs, your abdomen has to contract slightly. You can place your hand on your belly and feel it contract as you push the air out. This deep-breathing technique is employed in most forms of yoga and as an adjunct to Zen, or the *kia!* grunt that martial art experts use when breaking a board. In Japan, the lower stomach is called the *hara,* and *hara* breathing is practiced as part of meditation to help calm the body and still the mind. In the Tibetan Buddhist tradition this is called "pot-shaped" breathing because that describes the distention of the diaphragm during this technique (perhaps explaining the appeal of the classic Buddha belly). In India, as with everything else related to psychophysical practices, yogic breathing has been refined to an art with many variations. One, known by its Sanskrit name of *ujjayi pranayama,* is particularly useful in calming the nerves and even inducing sleep.

The calming and rejuvenating receptors in the lower lobes trigger the parasympathetic nervous system and remind your body that life is not an emergency, so that you are sure to burn fat. Exercise has an effect on the lungs something like the way blowing up a balloon affects the elasticity of the rubber in the balloon. It forces the rib cage to open up so that even after you stop exercising, you are naturally breathing into those lower lobes of your lungs. And the best way to activate those lower receptors is to breathe through your nose.

The physical design of the nose makes use of turbinates, or bones shaped like spirals, with whorls or ridges decreasing in size from base to apex. These turbinates drive the air all the way down into the lower lobes of your lungs. This design was incorporated into modern gas, steam, and water turbines, like the ones in your car's motor that are engineered to drive the air efficiently through the engine. The initial design of the internal combustion engine utilized big valves that sucked air in much the way your mouth does. As air went into the piston, it mixed with gasoline, and the mixture was ignited by a spark plug in the piston chamber. The problem was that the mixture would always explode in the same place, and the car would wear out very quickly. Engineers then designed a valve that more closely resembled the turbinates in the human nose by swirling the air around and mixing with the gas all over the piston chamber. That kind of design, which is prevalent today, has extended the life of most engines and was the precursor to the turbocharger.

Based on simple physics, then, the nose is the desired organ for breathing and the mouth is the backup or emergency organ. If you saw a bear in the woods, for instance, you would take a quick upper-chest, gasping breath that would trigger the stress receptors—adrenal emergency hormones to get you up a tree, pronto! To our detriment, we have been conditioned to do this all day long so that our body is getting a message that life is an emergency 28,000 breaths a day. Since, as we now know, stress is the primary cause of such a high proportion of diseases, this is an unacceptable way to go through life. I will show you how you can learn to breathe into the lower calming, fat-burning lobes of the lungs all day long, activating a rejuvenating and pacifying experience 28,000 times each day. The best part is that the exercises I will show you are also a model for handling the stress in your life. If I can get you to handle high levels of exercise stress with a calming response, then you can learn to bring that experience into all aspects of your life so you can handle mental, emotional, and physical stresses with the same calm you can produce during exercise. It is the "eye of the hurricane" effect—the more often you can establish this neurological calm, the more productive you can be.

The horse, among the speediest animals on earth, is what is called an obligate nose breather, meaning it *must* breath through the nose because it cannot breathe through its mouth. Next to a horse's nostrils along the side of its head are six-inch turbines that swirl the air into a stream that is driven all the way into the deepest lower lobes of its lungs, several feet away. As infants, we, too, were obligate nose breathers. We did not know how to breathe through our mouths, but we learned as a response to stress. That first slap on the behind was traditionally used to stimulate the baby in some way and get it to cry; as a result of this overstimulation, infants took their first mouth breath. The stress response that triggers crying also elicits upper-chest breathing rather than the nose breathing that is natural to human infants.

Like burning sugar reserves for quick energy, mouth breathing is ideal *for emergencies*. But as a regular habit it has several notable drawbacks. To begin with, when babies have to breathe through the mouth, they cannot nurse. Mouth breathing then becomes identified in the infant's psyche with a lack of nourishment and security. Breathing through the mouth, especially at night, also tends to dry out the throat. The small hairs that line the nostrils serve to filter out impurities, and breathing through the mouth obviously bypasses this mechanism. Of course, you can't breathe only through your nose. The ideal is a balance between upper and lower lobe activity, between activating the sympathetic and parasympathetic nervous systems.

Lungs are delicate and the job of the stress receptors in the upper lobes is to handle pollutants, pollens, and irritants in emergency situations. If you're going to breathe into the lower lobes of your lungs, you need your sinuses and nasal passages, which have mucous membranes to filter and warm or cool the air, and small hairs called villi to help filter out dust and other impurities. When you drive the air all the way down into the lower lobes of the lungs, you not only activate between 60 and 80 percent of the blood supplies there, but you also push open the lower rib cage, helping it to become more flexible. Now instead of acting like a cage squeezing on your heart and lungs, your ribs can actually massage your heart and lungs 28,000 times each day. This will help prevent the stiffness and inflexibility of the rib cage that besets most people as they age and especially after a heart attack.

Although science says that the body seems to get oxygenated well enough with just the upper lobes of the lungs, that does not mean that the lower lobes are not necessary. In fact, I believe the lower lobes of the lungs help the body cope with stress and get rid of waste more efficiently without going into oxygen debt. The key to handling physical stress is how well the body removes carbon dioxide waste products, which is one of the responsibilities of the lungs. When people huff and puff while exercising hard, they are struggling to get rid of carbon dioxide. If you can't dispose of carbon dioxide and other waste products of the blood through the breathing process, those waste products will be pushed into your muscles, crystallize, and cause stiffness and soreness. This will also force the body into a constant fat-storing, sugar-burning emergency that has become a way of life for most Americans.

Whenever you exercise you produce lactic acid, which in normal circumstances is converted back into glycogen on the muscle site. But if the body is pushed too hard, it can't convert all that lactic acid. The brain wants to send the lactic acid back into the bloodstream and get rid of it through the respiratory and cardiovascular systems. But once that lactic acid gets into the bloodsteam, it goes back to your heart. Sensing too much toxic lactic acid, your heart perceives an emergency and starts beating faster, at the same time as you start to breathe faster. Those are the first signs that your body is going into a survival response, and that is what I want you to tune into so that you know exactly when you cross the line from a calming, energizing, oxygenating experience of exercise to an emergency.

We have been trained to exercise until we get to a place they call the blood lactate threshold, where we get the uncomfortable feeling of being pushed too hard. This is the point where you produce so much blood lactate (lactic acid) on the muscle site that this waste product reduces the flow of oxygen, resulting in an emergency. You then have to go into what's called anaerobic ("without oxygen") activity, which means that you can't process oxygen anymore. This is a full-blown emergency, your last gasp before you blow up. Conventional exercise wisdom says that it's okay if you exercise right up to that lactic acid threshold. Further than that and you go into a last-ditch emergency effort to keep running; but if you stay underneath that anaerobic threshold, you'll be able to exercise for a longer period of time.

Unfortunately, by the time you've gotten that close to the anaerobic threshold, you've already produced so much blood lactate that you've begun to break your body down. You're going to produce stress-fighting hormones and wind up with stiff, sore muscles. But if you can spot that emergency coming as soon as your breath starts to shorten, you can reset the breath rate to a slower rhythm and then begin to nurse your performance level higher and higher (as I will demonstrate in the next chapter). Over time you'll see the body proving very gracefully how much stress it can endure without responding to that stress as an emergency. You will now have the ability to distinguish the boundary between an emergency state and a calming state. Then if you cross the line from calm to emergency, at least it will be your choice. It's a little like the image of the balloon I used before. If you blow into that balloon really hard, you will probably burst it, whereas if you stretch the membrane first and then blow into it a little at a time, you can make it so elastic that you can inflate it to a much larger size.

Breathing through the mouth creates a great rush of oxygen into the upper lungs, but it also represents such a shock that the body cannot relax and open up the lower lobes—so the breath rate slows down. Some of Vedic texts say that people are limited in lifespan by the number of breaths they are allotted. Normally we use about 18 breaths per minute (bpm), but when we exercise, we may go up to as many as 50 or 60 bpm. If you have only a certain number of breaths and you can get your body to do the same amount of work at 14 bpm that most people are expending 50 bpm to do, that's a huge savings. The reason the body can handle more stress with slower breaths is that when you begin to open up those lower lobes of your lungs, the body can activate the oxygen-rich alveoli in the lower lobes of your lungs. Alveoli are tiny air sacs clustered at the end of the bronchioles that deliver oxygen to the lungs. The lungs have about 300 million such clusters, and wrapped around each alveolus are pulmonary capillaries, the smallest blood vessels in the lungs. This is where the vital exchange of gases takes place, as red blood cells expel carbon dioxide and absorb oxygen through the thin capillary and alveolus walls. It may take more time for the air to get to the alveoli in the lower lobes, and more time to exchange oxygen and CO_2, but it's so much more efficient that you don't have to breathe as rapidly or take in as much air. You won't pant and puff the way you do during an emergency, when you're struggling to get air in and get waste out. The body can breathe in slowly, make a much more efficient exchange, and get rid of the waste in a more relaxed and efficient fashion—activating the calming nerves along the way.

The difference is clear when you watch someone huffing and puffing so hard that the person is hyperventilating—a real stress response. Some people think that's a good sign, because if you're breathing hard you must be working hard, and you're really going to burn some calories! Not so. If you see somebody on the phone constantly screaming and ranting, you wouldn't necessarily think the person was a good executive or was getting a lot of work done. But the Western mindset sees merit in the need to push and struggle. As a result we end up exhausted, fatigued, with chronic disease, and, more important than anything else, not enjoying our lives.

BREATHING FOR STRESS REDUCTION

We saw that springtime resets the body for fat metabolism so that when you get to summer you aren't overwhelmed by all the carbs and sugars being harvested. In much the same way, breathing as I've been prescribing provides you with a baseline of stress-handling ability that allows you to cope with all kinds of stress in your life without blowing up and triggering cravings for emergency fuel, namely sugar. The body was designed with layers of prevention built in to handle increasing layers of stress.

But we have overruled so many of these layers of natural prevention that we are beginning to experience the direct impact of stress on our nervous system in a way that was never supposed to happen.

In traditional cultures parents would watch their children sleep and make sure they were breathing correctly, actually training them how to breathe. If a mother saw a child lying on its back with its mouth wide open, she would turn it on its side, tuck in its chin, and squeeze its lips shut to gently force the baby to breathe through its nose rather than its mouth. We have almost totally lost this art, which helped prevent colds and fostered proper respiratory development.

When I work with patients who suffer from chronic sinus irritation, allergies, or a deviated septum, I sometimes suggest a commercial product called Breathe Right to enhance their ability to increase oxygen intake and CO_2 production. Breathe Rights look like butterfly bandages; when affixed across the bridge of the nose they help to expand the nostrils and increase the diameter of the nasal passages. (You may have noticed some pro football players wearing them because, with their protective mouthpieces inserted, they need all the help they can get in breathing through the nose.) These little aids are not a cure-all, but scientific studies have shown that they increase respiratory efficiency by 30 percent. If you use them while exercising, they help give you an idea of what it can feel like to breathe the way we were intended to. The more you breathe through your nose, the easier and more natural it becomes. You might even practice doing so at night as you lie in bed waiting to fall asleep. Consciously keep your mouth closed and take long, slow breaths through your nose. You might try putting on a Breathe Right before you retire to get the proper feeling. Once the sinuses open up to this breathing experience, you will not need Breathe Rights; breathing through the nose will feel normal after a while.

Breathing through your nose sets in motion a chain reaction of good results. You draw more oxygen deeper into the lungs. At the same time you are pushing your rib cage open so that it becomes more flexible, and when that happens you naturally begin to breathe more deeply through your nose during the day without thinking about it. If this sounds like the impossible dream to you, just consider my own history.

Fifteen years ago, when I first started this approach to breathing dur-

ing exercise, I had a deviated septum, a broken nose, and chronic allergies. I had just come back from India, where I had learned the value of
nose breathing, and I began teaching some small classes about the technique. People were coming up to me after a couple of weeks and saying,
"Wow! This is fantastic! I can't believe how I feel!" But I was having so
much trouble breathing through my nose that I couldn't relate to them.
I knew that theoretically it was a good idea, but I just couldn't experience it. When I went for a run, it required so much strain to not breathe
through my mouth that my cheeks and lips would go numb. My mouth
would get exhausted from my squeezing it shut for so long. Meanwhile,
I was producing so much mucus that I was constantly having to stop and
blow my nose while exercising. I couldn't get any air at all through my
left nasal passage. It took me a year to blast through all the blocks to
breathing through my nose. Then one day, after finally teaching myself
to breathe this way during my workouts—just to increase the efficiency
of my exercise—I was walking in a mall with my wife when she pointed
out to me that I had involuntarily begun to breathe deeply through my
nose. All of a sudden what had seemed so unnatural felt normal. In the
beginning, it may not feel natural to you either, and you may think you
are going to choke or suffocate. But soon the naturalness of proper
breathing will assert itself and you will have established an entirely new
level of respiratory efficiency. I was a tough case; most folks get this
down in a couple of weeks.

DARTH VADER TO THE RESCUE

Now that you've heard about the benefits of nose breathing over mouth
breathing, it's time to experience the difference firsthand. Sitting up in
a relaxed posture but with your spine straight, inhale a big, full breath
through your mouth. Then exhale, breathing only through your mouth,
and repeat this sequence three times. Now take the same number of deep
full breaths but breathe only through your nose. As you repeat these
cycles, pay attention to the differences. Having worked with thousands
of people on this experiment, I can report the most common responses.
The first is that because nasal passages are narrower, it takes longer to
breathe through the nose than through the mouth, but the nasal breath

also feels deeper and more relaxed. Ultimately you may feel calmer and more centered after breathing only through the nose for several minutes. Breathing through the mouth is obviously easier, but the breaths tend to feel more shallow, involving only the upper chest. If you are taking big breaths as suggested, you may have a tendency to feel dizzy because of the hyperventilation effect, and your mouth and throat may get dry and irritated.

The first question you may be asking is whether you need to learn a technique simply to be able to breathe through your nose while exercising. Even if you don't normally breathe through your nose all day, you *could* if you had to, right? Well, let's see. Can you close your mouth, breathe only through your nose, and do a moderately brisk walk or a moderate run for at least 20 minutes without having to breathe through your mouth? Try it, and if you can't do it, then move on to the second step.

Go for a walk and breathe deeply in and deeply out through your nose, counting how many steps you take for one full inhalation and exhalation combined. For example: 1, 2, 3 steps for the in breath; 1, 2, 3, 4 steps for the out breath, for a total of 7. I want you to keep trying to expand that number until you get to 21 steps total for one in breath and one out breath. How the numbers break down doesn't matter; it could be 6 in and 15 out. In the end, your exhale will probably be longer than your inhale, but it might take you some time to get there, so don't worry about it.

Once you've mastered that (it should take just a day), you're ready to try a relatively simple breathing technique that was developed thousands of years ago in India and is often used to help calm down or prepare for sleep. Its ancient Sanskrit name is *ujjayi pranayama*, but I have developed my own variation that I prefer to call "Darth Vader breathing" because of the sound it makes. There are several different ways to learn how to breathe like this. But adhering to my Golden Rule, if you don't feel comfortable making this sound or you're not sure how to do it, then don't bother. Just breathe through your nose the best you can.

Begin by closing your mouth and inhaling deeply through the nose; then, rather than exhaling through the nose, make a sound as if you were snoring, pushing the air to the back of your throat. It is not a vocal sound but more like the air resonating as if you were breathing through a respirator. You will exhale the air, but you won't feel it passing through your nose. It is, of course, since with your mouth closed there is nowhere else for it to go. You will hear a sound a little like Darth Vader's amplified breathing. You should also notice your stomach muscles contracting slightly, because if you're doing this correctly, you can't make the sound without slightly contracting your abdomen. The more you contract those abdominal muscles, the more pronounced the Darth Vader sound will be.

If you're not sure you have it, take a pair of sunglasses and blow on them with your mouth open, as if to fog them for cleaning. That *haaa* sound you make will come from inside your throat. Now close your mouth and gently make the same sound from your throat again. This time the air will be forced out through your nose but will actually feel like it is coming out through your throat—as if you were breathing through a tube in your esophagus. Once you get the knack of making the Darth Vader sound with short, shallow breaths, you can begin making longer, slower, and deeper exhalations, and you can make the sound during your inhalations as well. You need to use the Darth Vader breathing only during exercise, not all day. It is a remarkably useful calming technique, however, and you can use it while driving or before public speaking to help yourself relax.

Continue to be aware of your abdominal muscles expanding on the inhale and contracting on the exhale. The abdominals are the secondary muscles of breathing and respiration, but almost nobody uses them, since most of us breathe through our chest, rib cage, and collarbones. As a result, we end up stressing our trapezius muscles and holding on to stress in our neck and shoulders. We were never designed to breathe from there, and if your upper shoulders are squeezing to lift your rib cage so you can suck in air all day long, those muscles are going to be overworked and will become tense. When they're tense and tight they don't move in as much blood or move out as much waste as they should. When muscles lose blood, they lay down a kind of a tissue that doesn't need blood, called scar tissue or fibrous tissue. It's a little like the grass in a desert: When it is not getting enough water, the grass either gets tough or dies. In the same way, when the muscles are not getting enough blood, they grow tough and inflexible.

Scar tissue renders the shoulder muscles inelastic, and in time those muscles lose their ability to expand and contract. After years of unrelieved stress, the same thing happens to muscles all over your body, particularly around your ribs, until by the time you're 50, 60, 70, or 80 years old you can't touch your toes anymore. Eventually the rib cage becomes a literal cage, locking in and squeezing on the heart and lungs. As the joints themselves become stiff and rigid, they grow arthritic and painful. Strange as it may sound, the antidote for stress, stiffness, and arthritis is learning how to breathe properly. Breathing into the lower lobes of the lungs means you won't depend on only your upper neck and shoulders to draw air into the upper chest. That allows the trapezius and neck muscles to hold your head up, which is their original job.

Many of the muscles that support your lower back are also attached to the lower rib cage. So if your rib cage doesn't move, those connective muscles become rigid and stiff and rob the lower back of its flexibility. Think of a rope-and-pulley system, where the ropes are the muscles and the pulleys are the joints. Your rib cage then consists of 24 major pulley systems ranging along both sides of your twelve ribs, from the lower back to the neck and shoulders. If those pulleys are not moving, everything that attaches to the rib cage becomes more and more rigid. I've had patients call me up and say, "I've been following your breathing program and all of a sudden that pain in my foot is gone." Or their low-back pain is gone, or their neck and shoulder pain. I use this breathing technique clinically as a major part of my therapy with all my patients.

Many injuries are stress related because of a chain reaction: Stress creates tension; tension compromises blood supply; muscles get stiff and create pain. The solution is twofold:

1. Activate the neurological calm that doesn't let the muscles receive a message to tense up.
2. At the same time keep your rib cage flexible so that the joints remain supple and resilient.

When the diaphragm contracts during deep nasal breathing, it also squeezes onto the heart in what is called an abdominal diaphragmatic cardiac massage. This massage aids the heart in pumping while massaging waste away from the heart more efficiently. Even better, it activates the vagus nerve on the heart, which in turn activates the parasympathetic nervous system and tells the body that this is not an emergency. The more we can activate the vagus nerve, the more stress we can handle in our lives without a degenerative stress response. The idea again is to maintain the eye of the hurricane: The calmer you can keep your nervous system under stress, the more productive you can be.

This breathing exercise is a powerful model for handling the stress in our lives. In some of my original research, I measured brain waves during exercise with and without this breathing technique. Graph A shows typical brain wave activity during an alpha state, a calming response in the brain usually seen during sleep, meditation, or a relaxation technique. In Graph B the brain is in beta activity, the stressed and somewhat scattered state in which most people live their lives. Graph B is the typical picture of one of our subjects exercising without correct breathing. In Graph A the same subject used our breathing techniques and went into submaximal exertion, reproducing the same brain waves and calm you would get in a relaxation or meditation state. Imagine running as fast as you can while your brain responds to the experience as if you were sleeping or meditating. This is much like the experience or "runner's high" that athletes talk about when they are performing at their peak yet feel they are running slowly or with great equanimity. (I go into more detail about how to make this work during sports in my book *Body, Mind and Sport*.)

Graph A is an accurate rendering of what I have been calling the eye of the hurricane. If you can produce this calm while exercising, why not have it all day, 28,000 breaths a day? You are going to breathe this many times anyway, so by putting some effort into relearning how to breathe you can retain this calm response all day without even thinking about it. Once the rib cage becomes more flexible and resilient, you will find that you naturally breathe into the calming lower lobes all the time.

GRAPH A

BRAIN WAVE ACTIVITY DURING NASAL BREATHING EXERCISE

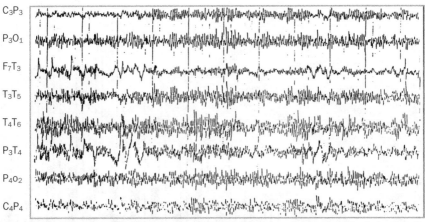

Alpha activity 11 minutes into "Listening Phase" (during bicycle ergometer submaximal stress test).

GRAPH B

BRAIN WAVE ACTIVITY DURING MOUTH BREATHING EXERCISE

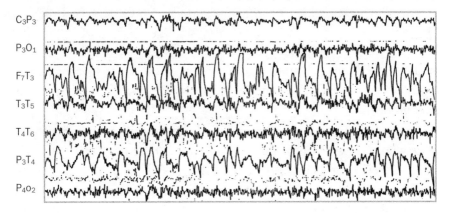

Exercise will force the rib cage open and then you can naturally have access to the this antistress influence all day long.

I believe this to be one of the most powerful stress-prevention techniques we have. It is a more powerful and constant influence even than spending an hour a day in meditation, yoga, or stress-reduction classes.

GRAPH C

PERCEIVED EXERTION MOUTH VS. NASAL BREATHING

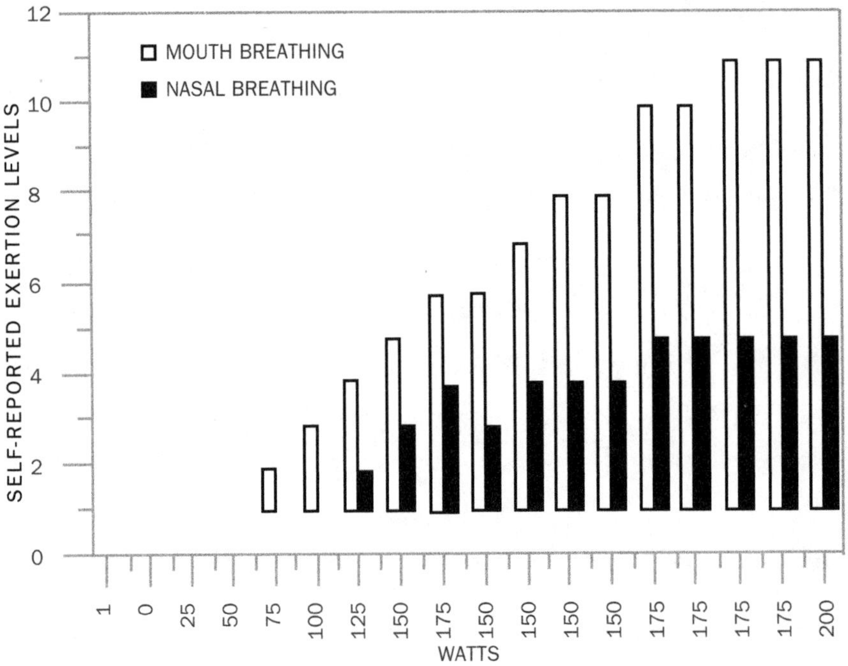

Although those are all fine, it makes more sense to me to activate the body's own constant, automatic stress preventer—the quality of your breath.

Graph C is a perceived exertion chart showing the responses of subjects who were asked how they felt during exercise on a scale of 0–10, with 10 being the worst. When the subjects did conventional exercise and the brain was stressed, they perceived the exertion as a 10—the worst they could feel. When they redid the exercise using the proper breathing technique as I instructed them, the brain when into a calm, eye-of-the-hurricane condition known as an alpha state (Graph A). When the brain was calm, the subjects performed the same amount of work, but their perception of the work was a 4 rather than a 10. Imagine coming home from work and instead of feeling as if you had been pushed to your limits and hitting a 10 on the chart, you felt as if you had pushed yourself to only a 4.

We can learn to handle stress in our lives by teaching our body not to respond to normal situations as emergencies. If we are convinced that bears are chasing us all day, we will have to activate the survival response all day long. Whereas with a little effort, you will find that the best way to handle stress and make sure your body burns fat is to spend a couple of weeks relearning how to breathe. And that is precisely what I will show you how to do in the following chapter.

CHAPTER 11

The Perfect Weight-Balancing Workout

AS A FORMER TRIATHLETE in the 1980s, I was well versed in how to "kill" myself during exercise. The "no pain, no gain" credo was in full swing and nobody wanted to hear that less is more. I thought I had reached my limit when I started getting dizzy, but my triathlon colleagues convinced me that this was a sure sign that I was reaching new heights in my training, and that it was just a phase I had to go through to become a better athlete. After a couple of acupuncture sessions to relieve the dizziness, I went back to training at full tilt. The problem was that I never improved beyond a certain point, no matter how hard I trained. It was clear that my body was limited by the amount of stress I could endure, and pushing beyond it just brought exhaustion, premature injuries, and a dread of my next workout. If I didn't have a race scheduled, I did not train. The things I once loved to do more than anything else—to swim, bike, and run—had become a chore. I wasn't improving; I was constantly fatigued and I began to question the benefits of this kind of intense exercise.

Years later I was invited to Moscow to help teach some of their coaches and athletes how to train less and accomplish more. The Russian coaches were complaining that to keep their athletes at a competitive level, they had to train so hard that they would get injuries and develop asthma or chronic colds throughout the season. The body responds to mental, physical, or emotional stress with the same degenerative chemistry. Cortisol levels rise, disease-producing free radicals are created, the body craves sugar, insulin and cholesterol levels increase, and the body stores fat—just to mention a few. If our bodies are convinced that all aspects of our lives are an emergency, and the above chain reaction becomes a constant part of life, whether while exercising or driving your kids to preschool, then we are in trouble.

The weight-balancing exercise program I'm about to lay out is designed to use exercise as a model to reeducate your body to metabolize fat, not sugar, as its main source of fuel. It is also designed to teach you how to handle more stress without triggering the body's degenerative stress response. As this happens, exercise will no longer be a "workout" you dread but an effortless experience you will look forward to each day. If you follow this program you will find that the calm you create during exercise also develops your ability to create calm when confronted by stress in your daily life. Soon you will be a fully mature hurricane possessing the ability to handle astonishing amounts of stress—whether mental, physical, or emotional—with an internal sense of peace and calm. You will come to realize that there is nothing you cannot handle.

THE BEST TIME TO EXERCISE

In chapter 4, I explained that the spring is the start of nature's new year, the time to plow the fields and plant the crops and spring into activity after a long winter's rest. I pointed out that in spring, nature is harvesting a low-fat diet to force our bodies into fat metabolism so as not to be overwhelmed by the high-sugar harvest of summer. In the same way that spring is the start of the new growing year, sunrise is the start of each period of daily growth. For the first four hours after sunrise, according to one Soviet study, the body's muscles grow stronger; this is the springtime of each day.

Just as the body is encouraged to burn fat in the spring, it is encouraged to burn fat after sunrise. If you don't utilize and move the muscles during this time, by 10:00 A.M. the body's fat stores will remain tucked away and you will reach for the easy fuel of sugar instead, craving a coffee break, doughnuts, chips, colas, and sweets. But if you use this time to move properly without triggering a sugar-burning emergency, the body will mobilize its fat stores as nature designed. You will feel revitalized with a much more stable baseline of energy throughout the day.

The nine-posture routine (Five-Minute Fat-Burning Workout) that I will describe on pages 224–230 can take 2 to 10 minutes and is a great fat-burning way to start each day. A few minutes every morning isn't a lot to ask, given the high energy levels, absence of inappropriate cravings, and dramatic feelings of well-being that will result. When you have more time—anywhere between 10 and 30 minutes or more—use the weight-balancing workout I am about to lead you through as well. This is best done before breakfast. I realize that right now this may feel like the worst time of day for many of you to exercise, but as we continue to bring your weight and breathing into balance with the natural rhythms of each day, your feelings will change. For years I was a confirmed night person and would never consider exercising in the morning. I always exercised at night after work. Now I don't start my day without at least doing the nine-posture routine or a weight-balancing workout that can last from 10 minutes to an hour, depending on how I feel and how much time I have. What used to feel totally unnatural—exercising in the morning—now feels like the only way to start my day. If a morning exercise session is impossible for you, then the second-best time is just after sunset, which usually means after work. Midday workouts are all right, although far from ideal, but should not in any way interfere with your mealtime.

If you feel you can't work out in the morning because you're simply too stiff to move, don't give up yet. I'm going to start this weight-balancing workout with a series of movements just about anybody can do. You can literally crawl out of bed onto your hands and knees and be in perfect position to start this workout.

Before we start, though, let's review the breathing we discussed in the last chapter. Begin with deep nasal breathing on the in and out breath. If you feel a little dizzy from this, it is not hyperventilation, which is an openmouthed panting reaction to stress. This nasal breathing lightheadedness is usually the result of having an unaccustomed amount of oxygen or blood going to your brain. For most people, it goes away naturally in a few hours or a couple of days, so work on the deep nasal breathing until you can do it for 5 minutes without any lightheadedness. If you get dizzy or feel winded, just stop and take a few regular breaths, then resume breathing a little less deeply through the nose. Once you've got that down, add the Darth Vader breath only on the exhale, until you can do this for 5 minutes without any problem. If you need to, take a moment now to review the Darth Vader technique from chapter 10.

DARTH VADER BREATH REVIEW

EXHALE: MAKE THE Darth Vader sound with complete exhale, starting with the upper chest and working down, finally squeezing your belly to get rid of every last bit of air from the lower lobes of your lungs.

Inhale: The inhale is the reverse of the exhale. First fill the lower lobes of your lungs (belly), then the middle and upper lobes. After you take in as much air as you can through your nose (no Darth Vader sound on the inhale), start the Darth Vader exhale.

Once you feel comfortable with nasal breathing and the Darth Vader sound, proceed with the following series of stretching exercises specifically designed to open up your rib cage and make it more flexible. They are taken from yoga principles that help you activate the lower lobes of the lungs more easily. The key is to be able to have access to the lower lobes not only while you exercise but all day long, automatically, the way it is supposed to happen.

STRETCHING THE RIB CAGE

STEP ONE

Spend 5 or 10 minutes with the following succession of upward-downward, dog-type stretches (fig. 1). Each position is linked to the next with the breath, so try to stay conscious of your breathing throughout to maintain the rhythm. Inhale as deeply as possible through the nose, and exhale using the Darth Vader sound—or, if you feel uncomfortable making this sound, just squeeze out each exhale as thoroughly as possible with a regular nasal breath. As you exhale you will be flexing your body; when you inhale you will be extending your body. This flexion and extension of the rib cage and the spine while breathing maximally will force the rib cage and spine to open up and become more flexible. Flexibility is crucial if you are eventually to gain access to the lower lobes of the lungs and with them, the calming nerves and the oxygen-rich blood.

During this series of stretches, you'll need to set a rhythm for your breath that you will maintain throughout the rest of your workout. Set this rhythm to breaths as deep as possible, and become aware of this rhythm as you continue to stretch, because in a little while I will ask you to use this rhythm to monitor how fast and hard you are working. If this rhythm shortens during exertion, it means that you are going too fast and you should slow the pace and reset the breath rate to its original slow, deep, and long rhythm.

STEP ONE STRETCHING ROUTINE

Note: During all these positions, how deeply you breathe is much more important than how perfectly you execute the position. The key is to use the breath to create flexibility in the rib cage.

POSITION ONE: While on all fours, exhale completely, squeezing out as much air as possible as you arch your back into the air. Tuck your head gently as you round your entire spine. Use the Darth Vader sound with all exhale flexion positions if comfortable.

POSITION TWO: While in the same position on all fours, start the inhale as you raise and extend your head and let your belly button go toward the floor. Take in as much air as possible as you arch your spine in the opposite direction from Position One. Inhale on all positions *without* the Darth Vader sound, but as deeply as possible through the nose.

POSITION THREE: Repeat Position 1

POSITION FOUR: Sit back on your heels and reach for the sky with your arms and hands as you inhale as deeply as possible, stretching and lengthening the spine.

POSITION FIVE: Keeping your arms over your head in the same plane with your spine, slowly bend at the waist and bring the spine, head, and arms to the ground at the same time. Feel the stretch in your lower back and breathe out as deeply as you can (with Darth Vader sound), squeezing out every last bit of air.

POSITION SIX: Repeat Position Four

POSITION SEVEN: Repeat Position One

POSITION EIGHT: Repeat Position Two

POSITION NINE: Repeat Position Five

POSITION TEN: Slowly lunge forward and lie on your stomach with your hands in a push-up position. Take a long, deep inhale through your nose as you pull your chest off the floor, using your back muscles to pull the spine into extension. Try not to use your arms to push up.

POSITION ELEVEN: Push back into Position Five as you exhale deeply

POSITION TWELVE: Repeat Position Ten

POSITION THIRTEEN: Repeat Position One

POSITION FOURTEEN: Repeat Position Two

POSITION FIFTEEN: Tuck your toes and push up onto all fours, stretching your buttocks as high as they will go. Try to keep your arms straight and your heels to the floor as best you can as you exhale deeply.

POSITION SIXTEEN: Repeat Position Two

POSITION SEVENTEEN: Repeat Position One
Note: You can combine this series of positions in any way you like. Some people who are just starting out can do only Positions One and

STEP ONE STRETCH ROUTINE

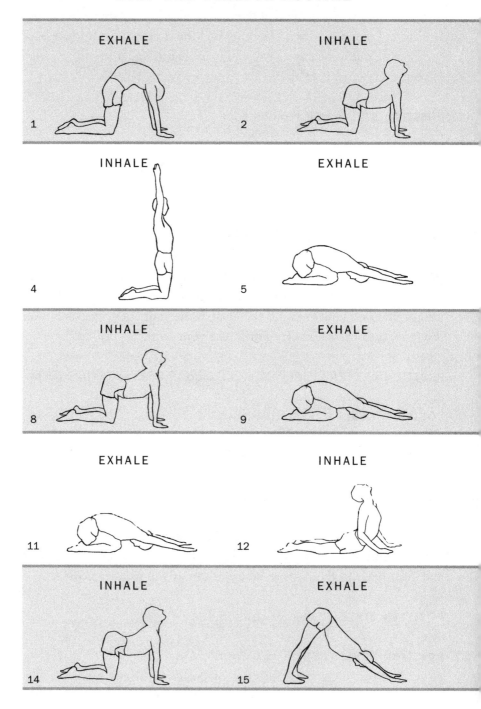

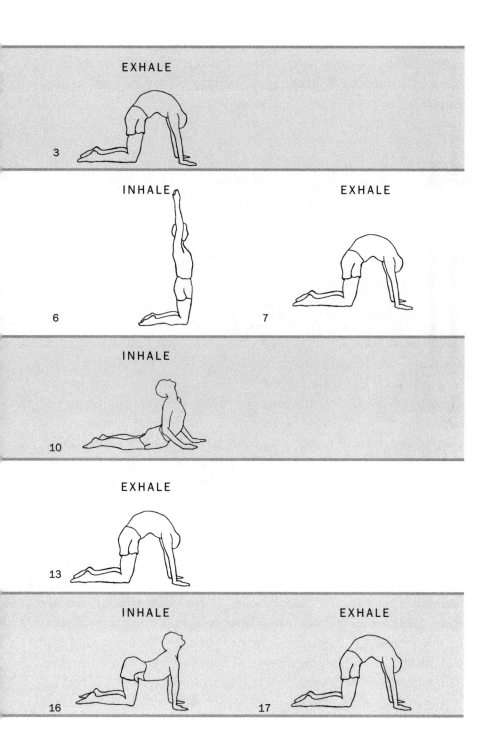

Two over and over. That is perfectly fine, because you will soon find that you are stronger and more flexible and can add more positions from this routine. When the entire series is easy for you, move on and try the Five-Minute Fat-Burning Workout (nine postures) described later in this chapter.

STEP TWO

Once you have finished stretching and have set the rhythm of your breath, start walking for about 5 to 10 minutes, breathing ridiculously deeply in and out, so that you are actually exercising your lungs while you're walking. Keep the same rhythm in your breath from the stretching exercises in Step One while walking. Count your steps as I showed you in chapter 10, keeping track of the total number of steps during the in and out breaths combined.

The goal here is to perfuse all of the lobes of your lungs, activating as much of those lower lobes as you can. Before you start any exertion, make sure to get as much access to that oxygen-rich, calming region as possible. That's why the main point of Step Two is to walk slowly and breathe deeply. This is the hardest part of the workout, because breathing deeply takes some getting used to if you have never done it before. If you've ever had any training in yoga, meditation, the martial arts, or even natural childbirth, you've probably learned to breathe this way for brief periods of time. In any case, depending on how relatively obstructed your nasal passages are, it requires a certain amount of persistence. So be prepared to feel as if you don't actually want to breathe so deeply! That's part of reeducating your rib cage so that you'll still be able to touch your toes when you're 80 years old.

Let me emphasize again how important it is during this part of the workout to tune in to the rhythm of the breath as you maximally inhale and exhale through your nose. Use the Darth Vader exhale if you are comfortable with it, because it will enhance the calming effects of regular nose breathing. Depending on your fitness level, you may find that you can still accomplish the mission of Step Two with a slow jog rather than just a slow walk. The point is to exercise slowly enough and breathe deeply enough to get as much access into those lower lobes of the lungs as possible.

EXERCISE TIP

A S YOU BREATHE deeply and walk slowly during this part of the workout, you will notice a comfortable space between each breath. You are not holding your breath to make this space, but because you are walking slowly and the exertion is minimal, you will experience a natural lack of urgency to take the next breath. Tune in to and maintain this space between each breath, because as we begin to walk faster in Step Three and the breath grows more shallow, that comfortable space will be the first thing to go. Losing this space will be your monitor of how stressful the exercise is becoming.

STEP THREE

While maintaining the same rhythm of the breath you had in Steps One and Two, start to walk faster. At some point the rhythm of your breathing, which you set up in the very beginning and locked in while you were walking slowly and breathing deeply, will start to pick up. As you begin to exercise more intensely, you will eventually open up your mouth involuntarily, out of sheer survival instinct, and take a big, old-fashioned, gasping mouth breath, the kind you would take if a bear were chasing you. That's your emergency breath, and it's perfectly natural at this stage of the game. But now we're trying to learn to anticipate the emergency before it arrives. So as soon as your breath—we're talking nose breathing with Darth Vader exhales here—goes from long and slow and deep to that first hint of shortening up and losing the space between each breath, that's your indication that the emergency is coming. At that point, slow down your walk and revert to your original breath rate.

STEP FOUR

Once you reset that rhythm, try to walk faster again. But this time when you walk faster, you should find that you can beat your previous score—increasing the number of steps you can take during one complete in and out breath. Even though you'll be walking faster, you'll still be breathing at the same depth, or even slower. As soon as you walk a little bit too fast and your breath starts to shorten up, back off again. Return to your original walking speed, reset your original breath rate, and then pick up the pace again. Each time you increase your pace, your body will let you do a little bit more work with the same amount of effort. You just keep returning to your old starting point and going back up again, and you keep improving your old score. In the process, you are teaching your body how to handle stressful situations, with exercise as a model for stress. Each time you reset your original speed and breath rate and work up to your limit—to the point where you lose that space between breaths—back off and repeat the process, improving the amount of work you can handle each time. If you have to take a big emergency mouth breath, you have gone too far. Always try to stop just before you get there, reset your original breath rate, then work back up again. Soon you'll be doing more work—handling more stress—with the same neurological response you had at rest.

As you melt down each barrier of stress, your body emerges with a new barrier at a higher level. When you're nearing that higher level and your breath wants to shorten up in the emergency response, you will push to get more air, but you will also be pushing that air into the lower lobes of your lungs, forcing them open. When you revert to the easy part of the workout again, you make your gains permanent.

In keeping with my principle of paddling downstream, you will make your permanent gains when there's no stress on your system. That's when you can breathe easily into what you were previously pushing into as you were working harder. Now you can set up a new rhythm at a deeper level of the lower lobes, then take that deeper level of the lower lobes, then take that deeper level into higher levels of work. The deeper you go, the more oxygen you get and the more you improve your exchange of oxygen and CO_2 and your activation of calming nerves. You will slowly discover that you can handle higher levels of stress and that the barrier you had a minute ago is now melting down to a higher level of work.

Stick with the back-and-forth rhythm until you can feel the results. You can easily do this by taking a 20- or 30-minute walk and monitoring your breathing levels as you go, counting your steps for each in-and-out breath. Make it your long-term goal to reach 21 steps for one complete inhale and exhale combined.

STEP FIVE: A TEST RIDE

If you want to try it out a little more scientifically, go to a gym that has a treadmill and follow this procedure. After you've done the stretches from Step One, set the treadmill on 2½ to 3½ miles an hour at zero degrees elevation. Walk slowly on the treadmill and breathe in and out as deeply and slowly as you can for 10 minutes. (Ridiculously deeply in, ridiculously deeply out.)

Next, keeping your speed at whatever is comfortable for you (2½ to 3½ mph), increase the elevation by 1 degree every 15 seconds. Along the way ask yourself, "Am I breathing with the same rhythm as I climb this hill that I had at zero degrees elevation?" As you begin to walk faster or up a steeper hill, the breath rate will insidiously increase on you. That is why it is so important to pay close attention to the rhythm of the breath. Remember to listen for that space between each breath as a monitor of how well you are staying in the eye of the hurricane. As soon as you start breathing faster and the space disappears, you have lost the calm eye of the hurricane and are triggering an emergency response unecessarily.

At 4 degrees, let's say, you will feel your breath starting to be a bit labored. Go back to zero degrees elevation, reset your breathing, and get the rhythm going, this time making it even deeper. Once you have caught your breath, go up again 1 degree every 15 seconds. This time you should be able to go up past 4 to 5, 6, or 7 degrees before your breath feels labored. Once again return to zero degrees, keeping the speed at 2½ to 3½ miles an hour, wherever it is.

Once back at zero degrees, reset the breath to an even deeper, longer, and slower rate. After 1 to 3 minutes of this, depending on how long it takes you to get your comfortable breath back, go up again, this time to 8 or 9 degrees elevation and then back to zero when the breath shortens up. Let your breath return to baseline or deeper, then run the elevation up to 10 or 11 degrees, 1 degree every 15 seconds. At 10 or 11 degrees you should begin to approach the emergency state. Don't wait for that to happen, slow down, set up a new breath rhythm, and then begin increasing the elevation again. By the time you get up to 12 or 13 degrees, you're going up such a steep hill that it makes more sense to go back to zero degrees and then increase your speed, maybe from 4 to 5½ mph. Get a stable deep breathing rhythm and start the elevation process again.

If you came to one of my classes, you might expect to go from 4 degrees to 11 degrees on your first workout. Within 15 minutes you would be doing three times as much work as you had been at the beginning, and would prove to yourself that you can breathe in a totally different way. You would immediately understand that with this program you are teaching your body how to handle stress–any kind of stress–without responding to that exertion as an emergency. Most people show great improvement within the first workout. Although the improvements are small, they are continuous. Over two or three workouts you should see marked progress, and within a few short weeks you will be receiving very nice dividends in terms of health benefits and enjoyment of your exercise. Ironically, those people who are already fit often have to back off and start much slower than they are used to doing. They can become frustrated in the beginning because they have to open up their rib cage just like anyone else. This takes some time and patience and requires the ability to learn how to listen to your body, rather than stoically overruling it and driving it to exhaustion the way we have been taught. But in the end you will increase fitness levels without breaking your body down in the name of building it up, losing weight, or looking good. As I've said throughout, life is all about how much you can handle without going into survival mode. How big is your eye of the hurricane, and as a result how powerful can your winds of energy become? Too often we try to create a lot of wind with no hub of composure and calm. All that will result is a little tropical storm that blows itself out before gaining strength.

Properly understood, what I have just given you is more than just a breathing technique. It's a practice for learning how to listen to your body and discern whether it is in an emergency situation or a state of calm. Once you learn how to do that, it becomes second nature. Your level of self-awareness will rise, and that is something you can apply to all kinds of situations, such as monitoring the moment when your sense of irritation boils over into anger or aggression, the moment when hunger becomes panic, or when fatigue becomes depression. This is not to say that you can't ever be in an emergency, but when you are, you'll be the first to know, and you'll also know that you don't have to stay there all day long. Now you can do something about it.

At the end of each workout, repeat the rib cage stretches from Step One or do the nine-posture Five-Minute Fat-Burning Workout on pages 225–230.

WEIGHT-BALANCING WORKOUT REVIEW

Step 1 Do the rib cage stretching exercises in figure 1. (5–10 mins.)

Step 2 Walk or run slowly with deep nasal breathing and Darth Vader exhale to set breathing rhythm. (5–10 mins.)

Step 3 Walk or run faster. As soon as breath shortens, slow down to original breath rate.

Step 4 Try to walk faster again, noticing that you can walk faster than before but still breathe with the same rhythm. When breathing shortens, slow down all the way and return to original breath rate.

Step 5 Keep repeating Steps 2, 3, and 4, resulting in deeper, longer, and slower breaths each time you return to Step 2. (10–20 minutes)

Step 6 Complete your workout with either Step 1 or the nine-posture sequence on pages 224–230.

Do this program for 20 to 30 minutes, three to four times a week, for maximum improvement.

FULL RESPIRATORY CAPACITY

Each time you do the Weight-Balancing Workout, you should keep two immediate goals in mind. The first is to perceive the difference between a mouth breath and a nose breath. Once you set the rhythm of the breath through the nose, listen for when your breath shortens or the mouth has to open during increased exertion. This is the first hint of an approaching emergency. It is crucial that you know when your body is calm and when it is perceiving an emergency.

The second goal is to notice that when you return to your original breath rate each time you go faster and the breath shortens, your body will allow you to do more work–that is, go faster before you approach an emergency response. As you continue to build the amount of work you can do without eliciting the emergency response, the body is being taught how to handle more stress with less effort. As the lower rib cage opens to allow this to happen, you will gain a more efficient oxygen exchange. Soon, as the workload increases, your body will find it more efficient under stress to breathe longer, deeper, and slower because it now understands this gives it access to the oxygen-rich lower lobes.

As you continue this workout for a few weeks, watch your breath as you increase your workout intensity. Your body's first response to more stress will gradually change from breathing faster and eventually gasping to breathing longer, deeper, and slower. Along the way, that deeper breathing will activate the calming nerves in the lower lungs, reinforcing the message to the nervous system that this stress can be handled without an emergency response. In Graph D (Breath Rate #2), you can see the breath rates of the same subject using my deep breathing techniques and conventional exercise techniques. As the workload increased with conventional exercise (Control), the breath rate rose up to 50 breaths per minute (bpm). When the subject learned how to breathe correctly, the breath rate did not surpass 14 bpm while doing vigorous exercise. Yet the average breath rate for someone at rest is only 18 bpm! Imagine running as fast as your legs can carry you and still taking 4 breaths per minute less than when you are standing at rest. This may sound unbelievable, but it simply shows how inefficiently we breathe most of the time.

LONG-RANGE GOAL

If you study the chart more closely, you'll see that as the workload approaches 200 watts of resistance, the breath rate under conventional techniques rises sharply to approach 50 bpm, but the breath rate using my technique actually slows down slightly. This is an example of respiratory efficiency. Under higher levels of stress and strain, the body chooses to breathe more slowly, and in doing so activates a calming response rather than the classic emergency or survival response. When

GRAPH D

BREATH RATE

MOUTH BREATHING VS. NASAL BREATHING EXERCISE

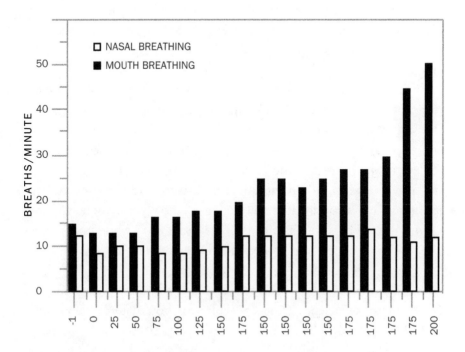

you exercise, watch your body's first response to stress. If your breath rate shortens, just follow the plan I laid out for you. But if the body's first breathing response is to breath longer and deeper and slower while increasing the workload, then your body is choosing to be more efficient under stress rather than immediately triggering the emergency response with shallower upper-chest breaths and eventually a mouth breath. When your body chooses to breathe deeper as you run or exercise harder, that means you have developed respiratory efficiency, and all you have to do at this point is maintain that efficiency. Once you get to this level of rib cage elasticity, you will not need to do the stretching before and after each workout; you will be able to jump into exertion quickly and breathe calmly and deeply.

The first time this happened to me, I had been struggling with nose breathing for quite a while because of my history of allergies, a broken nose, and a slightly deviated septum. One day I went for a run with a small group of runners who I knew were much faster than I was, particularly with my having to breathe through my nose. I decided to hold on to my nose breathing for as long as I could and see what happened. To my surprise, the faster I ran the slower I breathed. I couldn't believe the experience! It seemed as though I could run all day and as fast as I wanted and never get fatigued. This was my first glimpse of respiratory efficiency.

Such efficiency is a goal worth seeking, not so much because you can run faster but because it means that when you are confronted with a stressful situation, whether mental, emotional, or physical, your body will respond by creating a bigger sense of calm. Remember, the bigger the eye of the hurricane, the more powerful the winds. In my opinion, this is a stress-handling technique first and foremost, not an exercise technique. How you breathe will determine how you handle the stress in your life. When you start to become more calm while under stress, you will have tapped into your greater human potential.

FIVE-MINUTE FAT-BURNING WORKOUT

For respiratory efficiency to occur regularly in your daily life, your spine and rib cage need to be flexible and resilient. This is why doing the rib cage stretches on pages 211–215 is so important in making this experience a reality. I have also designed another set of stretching exercises that are slightly more advanced than the rib cage stretches, and with a couple of weeks' work, most people can master them. I designed these positions to balance all three body types, winter, summer, and spring. In the same way that the three seasons repeat themselves in the daily cycle and over the course of our lives, they repeat themselves in our body. For instance, your liver, skin, eyes, and digestion are more like summer. Your nervous system is quick moving and light, like winter. And springtime corresponds to the heavy part of the body that holds on to water–fat cells, muscle cells, bones, and sinews. The three seasons are designed to strengthen, support, emphasize, and cleanse three different aspects of the body. Winter types have very active nervous systems, summer types have plenty of heat and strong digestive systems, and spring types are heavier and tend to have larger frames and slower metabolisms. We all have a little of each of these qualities in us, so it is a good idea, whatever your type, to support the nervous system, digestion, and structure on a daily basis. Think of this exercise as a one-a-day vitamin for these systems of the body.

I have identified three postures each for winter, summer, and spring. I designed these postures for people who come to my classes, most of whom have little or no background in any kind of yoga, let alone advanced asanas. The postures do not require any special skill or stamina or any previous experience of yoga, yet are simple and effective for keeping the body young, vital, and flexible. These stretches are coordinated with a deep rhythm of breathing through the nose, preferably with the Darth Vader exhale.

The whole routine takes most people about 5 minutes to complete, although in time you can zip through it in 2 minutes or stretch it out to 10, depending on how many breaths you take with each posture and how many times you repeat the set of nine. The series is perfect first thing in the morning, because if you do not have the time for a full weight-balancing workout, it is important to do a little something every day. A few short minutes with these nine postures and you will feel that you have done something good for yourself. The cumulative benefits of doing these postures along with the weight-balancing workout are dramatic. Remember Figure 1 in chapter 10: The harder you push in exercise, the *less* fat you burn. In these exercises you will force the body gracefully into fat metabolism, which is the key to maintaining ideal weight and keeping your energy levels high all day long. If any of these stretches are too difficult, then do not strain yourself but use the rib cage stretches on pages 211–215.

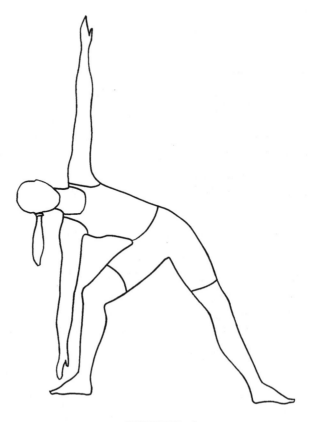

WINTER 1

Spread your legs a little farther apart than shoulder width with both feet pointing directly in front of you. Turn your right foot out about 60 degrees. Spread your arms out to the sides parallel to the floor. Take a big nasal in breath and bend forward toward the turned-out foot. Bring your hand to your ankle and hold that position. Or for a simpler version, rest your elbow on your knee, stay there, and take 3 deep nasal breaths with 3 big Darth Vader exhales. Raise your other arm over your head and stretch that arm up as far as it goes while you breathe. Repeat the procedure for the other side.

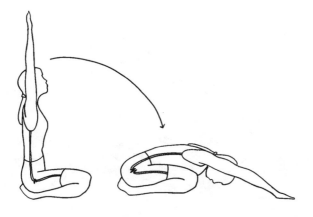

WINTER 2

From the Winter 1 position, drop to your knees and rest your buttocks on your heels. Reach for the sky with both arms and breathe in. As you exhale, bend over, collapse to the floor, and stretch your lower back. Go up and down 3 times, breathing in as you stretch up, and breathing out as you flex forward.

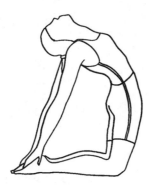

WINTER 3

While you are sitting on your heels and knees, reach back and grab your ankles, taking an in breath as you arch your back, and rise up while holding your ankles. Exhale as you come back to a neutral position. If you cannot reach your ankles, begin by placing your hands under your buttocks, then down to your heels as you develop more flexibility. Do this 3 times with 1 to 3 breaths each time.

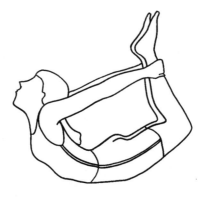

SUMMER 1

From this position lean forward and lie on your stomach. Reach back and grab you ankles, raise your head up, and pull your legs up as you inhale. Exhale as you lower them. Do this 1 to 3 times with 1 to 3 breaths.

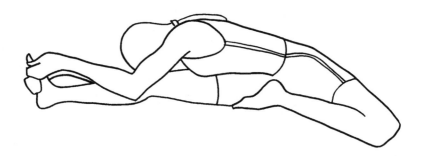

SUMMER 2

Now sit up and bring one foot into the crotch with the other outstretched. Take a big nasal in breath and reach for your ankle as you breathe out. Do this 1 to 3 times for each side.

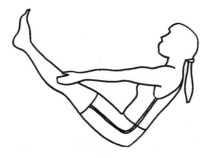

SUMMER 3

From this position raise your legs slightly apart and stretch out your arms so that your hands are almost touching your knees. Balance on your buttocks in this position so that your legs and torso form a V for 1 to 3 breaths. Your body may tremble slightly until you get the knack of this posture.

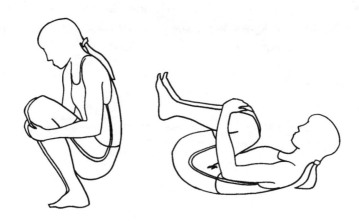

SPRING 1

From this balanced position, grab your knees and roll backward onto your back, pausing for a second or two. Then roll forward until your feet are flat on the ground but your body is still in the tuck position, and pause again for a second or two.

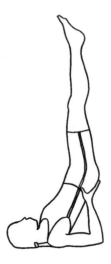

SPRING 2

From here roll up into a shoulder stand. Work up to this, and if you have any history of neck problems, get permission from your doctor to do this. If you cannot do a full shoulder stand, just roll back on your back from Spring 1 with your knees bent, support your back with your hands, and breathe one to three times.

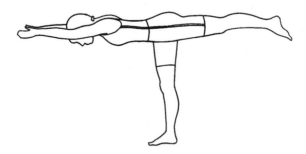

SPRING 3

Stand up and reach with both hands to the ceiling, then lean forward slightly while balancing on one leg, the other leg pointing straight out. Try to stay on this leg for 1 to 3 breaths. Repeat on the other leg.

Epilogue

THLETES ENGAGED IN RECORD-BREAKING compe-
titions have described the sensation of a "peak experience"
or being "in the zone," during which opposites of calm and
energy coexist effortlessly. At those moments, they say, they felt that
they were in slow motion while sprinting, or that they could see the
seams on a baseball coming toward them at 98 mph. When Roger
Bannister, the first person in recorded history to break the 4-minute
mile, was asked how he felt while accomplishing that feat he said, "I felt
no pain, no strain. I felt that the world seemed to be standing still. I felt
as if I was going slow!"

Whether running, eating, losing weight, fighting cravings, or in any
activity, when you are at your best and flowing downstream with the current, two things happen. First, the experience seems effortless; and second, your performance soars beyond your wildest dreams. I always use
these two indicators to monitor an accomplishment worth celebrating:
Was it fun? Was it effortless? Billie Jean King said that when she was at
her best playing tennis, she would transport herself beyond the turmoil
of the court to a place of peace and calm. Discovering that place is the
real goal of this book. If you can go there while eating, losing weight, in
your business, dealing with your family, and in all aspects of your life,
that is where you will also find happiness.

You now have all the information you need to get your weight down to your ideal level and keep it there without stress or strain. I've talked about many things in the course of this book, including seasonal harvests, nature's cycles, the importance of eating a big lunch, knowing your body type, and breathing properly, but the most important single thing to keep in mind is to avoid stress and strain in both eating and exercise. If you can keep your body from experiencing an emergency or survival situation regarding food and physical exertion, you will have gone a long way toward eliminating the most serious cause of weight gain. Of course, it helps to eat the appropriate foods for each season, to eat reasonable portions, and, as frequently as possible, to eat most of your food by mid-afternoon. But if you want to maximize your ability to maintain your ideal weight, then focus first on avoiding the perception of an "emergency" and everything else will follow from that.

When you like something you will stick with it; when it is a chore, you will eventually return to your initial behavior—but with an even lower opinion of yourself for having tried and failed yet again. What keeps us overweight and depressed also keeps us from achieving our full human potential. By that I don't just mean using more than the 3 percent of our potential brain function that scientists tell us we draw on. I am talking about achieving a level of happiness and satisfaction in your life that can never be taken away. This kind of contentment does not hinge on getting raises, owning a big house, or living the American Dream, the pursuit of which in so many cases has driven us to exhaustion and a sense of emptiness. Instead, your satisfaction will flow from the power of the universe itself. That's why I keep returning to the image of a hurricane, in which vast energies cycle around a core of calm and stillness. This powerful force of nature possesses what I consider the formula for human happiness, if only we will make use of it.

Stay in touch and let me know how it's going for you. The best way to reach me is through my Web site at www.lifespa.com

Good luck, and enjoy!

Appendix 1

GLOSSARY OF FOODS

Unless otherwise indicated, all protein, fat and carbohydrate amounts are based on 1 pound of each food.

ADZUKI BEANS (SEE LEGUMES)

AMARANTH

Native to ancient Mexico, amaranth is a gluten-free grain high in protein content. Harvested in late summer, it is ideal for building protein reserves in winter, and is a good alternative to wheat in spring, when wheat, which is high in gluten, is too heavy. Amaranth is also very high in the amino acids lysine and methionine, which make it a perfect and complete protein.

Best season: winter
Protein 19 g
Fat 6 g
Carb 6 g
(100 g)

APPLES

Typically harvested in the fall, apples have cooling properties that help the body cool and disperse the accumulation of summer's heat. Their high fiber content also helps to cleanse the intestines of impurities and heat and prepare the intestines for the dry winter to follow. Because of their astringent taste and cleansing properties, apples are also very useful in the spring. Apples and apple juice speed up the bowels and heal irritation while cleansing excessive mucus built up during the summer and winter months. If the mucus from breads, pastas, and dairy remains in the intestines all winter, it can dry up, become hardened, and cause constipation, malabsorption, and irritation or bleeding to the intestinal wall. Sweet and astringent in taste, apples are renowned for ameliorating intestinal ailments such as diarrhea and intestinal bleeding, which may result from excessive heat. Apples can be harvested all year long in dif-

ferent parts of the world, so eat sweet apples in the spring and summer
and sour apples in the winter. Although in general winter is not the best
time for apples, you may eat them cooked, sauced, or spiced with cinnamon. High in vitamins A and C and calcium.

Best season: summer
Protein 1.2 g
Fat 1.6 g
Carb 59.6 g

APRICOTS

Summer fruits that help cool the body from the summer's heat, apricots
are especially sweet and cooling when tree ripened, although in this state
they are rarely available in stores. The sour, unripe ones are all right in
winter, and dried apricots are good in the spring, as are all dried fruits.
Apricots are a laxative, they have anti-tumor properties, and, because of
high cobalt content, are good for anemia. They are also good for coughs
and fever.

Best season: summer
Protein 4.3 g
Fat .4 g
Carb 55.1 g

ARTICHOKES

Our word "artichoke" comes from a corruption of the Italian word for
pine cone, because it looks like one. Sweet, astringent, and cool, artichokes are harvested in summer and so are a great antidote for the summer's heat. They are also beneficial in the spring, and the heart of the
artichoke is good for winter. A good blood purifier, artichokes help fight
infections and have a very high alkaline content, making them both a
good spring cleanser and summer coolant. High in vitamins A and C,
iron, and calcium.

Best season: summer
Protein 5.3 g
Fat .4 g
Carb 19.2 g

ASPARAGUS

Harvested from February to July, asparagus is the perfect antidote for spring and summer. Bitter, sweet, astringent, and cool, it is extremely cooling and blood purifying. Because it is a diuretic that helps cleanse and strengthen the kidneys, a strong urge to urinate often arises after eating asparagus and the urine is often strong smelling. A blood cleanser and reproductive tonic, asparagus is good for edema, infections, skin disorders, and fever. A high alkaline food rich in chlorophyll to build red blood cells.

Best season: spring, summer
Protein 7.5 g
Fat .7 g
Carb 13.1 g

AVOCADOS

Consisting of 25 percent fruit oil, the highest of any fruit, avocados are sweet, warm, and heavy. Originally they came from the tropics and were harvested in the winter, making them the perfect antidote for mild tropical winters, as compared to, say, the fish oils that serve for insulation in Alaska's extreme winters. In the United States avocados are available year round but remain one of the best fruits to eat in the winter. They are also fine in the summer but too heavy for spring. Recent research has found three compounds in avocados that kill cancer cells. They are also good for blood and lungs and are high in copper and iron.

Best season: winter
Protein 7.1 g
Fat 55.8 g
Carb 21.4 9

BANANAS

Sweet and heavy when ripe, bananas have high fruit sugar that makes them good in the winter but a little too heavy in the spring. They are fine in summer, but if eaten in excess they can heat up the body. Unripe bananas are good for diarrhea and dysentery. Ripe, they are an excellent tonic for the muscular system because of their high potassium, and are good for anemia because of their high iron content. They are slightly heavy to digest and can be cooked or spiced with cardamom, ginger, or cinnamon.

Best season: winter
Proteins 3.6 g
Fats .6 g
Carb 69.9 g

BARLEY

Pearled barley is a low-gluten wheat alternative whose flour can be easily substituted for white flour in recipes. Primarily sweet and cool, it is best as a cooling antidote to the heat of summer. Barley holds two or three times its weight in water, giving it diuretic, kidney-strengthening, and anti-edema properties that make this grain useful in the spring as well as summer. As with all grains, it is indicated in moderation in the winter, but its dry nature makes it a poor winter choice in any event.

Best season: spring, summer
Protein 16 g (in one cup)
Fat 2 g
Carb 158 g

BEANS (SEE LEGUMES)

BEANS, GREEN

A cold early-spring crop harvested in April through June, beans are sweet and astringent. They are also diuretic and help move out the excess water of spring. High in natural fiber, they help to cleanse the liver and the blood, which makes them ideal for spring and summer.

Best season: spring
Protein 7.6 g
Fat .8 g
Carb 28.3 g

BEAN SPROUTS (SEE LEGUMES)

Sprouting dates back to ancient China, some 5,000 years ago. It is mentioned in the Bible, and early sailors survived on various kinds of bean sprouts. The most common are sprouted mung beans, but almost any bean, seed, or grain can be eaten in its sprouted form, including alfalfa, radishes, broccoli, and peas. Astringent and cool, sprouts are rich in vitamins and minerals, since all the nutrients for the adult plant are lively in the sprout. In some cases sprouts have been shown to have 300 to 600 times more nutrients than the adult plant or the original bean.

When mung beans are sprouted they have 600 percent more vitamin C and 300 percent more vitamin A than the bean itself. Given that statistic, eating one-half cup of sprouts would give you the equivalent of drinking six glasses of orange juice. Blood purifying and great for the liver, sprouts are a classic spring cleansing food because they are naturally sprouting during this season. During the sprouting process, they change from an acid winter food as a bean to an alkaline spring food. They are also great in the summer but if taken in excess they can be too cooling for winter.

Best season: spring
Protein   4 g (in one cup)
Fat   trace
Carb   7 g

BEEF
Sweet, heavy, and warm, beef is best eaten in the winter. In the spring and summer you should reduce heavy meats and eat them at the midday meal whenever possible. Traditionally, tribal people would not kill an animal for food if other foods were being harvested in abundance in the spring and summer. In the winter when food was scarce, animal protein intake would naturally rise.

Best season: winter
Protein   21 g
Fat   4 g
Carb   0 g
(2.4 oz. steak)

BEETS
Typically harvested in the fall, beets are great winter foods, as they are sweet and warm. In small amounts they are all right in spring as well but

are too heating for summer. Yet beet tops or greens are readily harvested all summer long to help cool the heat. Beets build the blood and cleanse the lymph and upper and lower digestive systems, are very high in vitamin A, and are demulcent for the dry winter months, meaning they soothe and protect mucous membranes. They also help bring on menstruation.

Best season: winter
Protein 5.4 g
Fat .3 g
Carb 32.6 g

BELL PEPPERS

Harvested late spring and summer, red, green, yellow, and purple bell peppers are sweet, astringent, and cooling for the summer months. They contain vitamin C equivalent to oranges, and high amounts of vitamin A and B make them useful for the immune system. In the winter, peppers are typically out of season and are too cooling unless baked and stuffed.

Best season: spring, summer
Protein 4.6 g
Fat .8 g
Carb 21.7

BITTER MELON

Originally harvested throughout Asia, China, and India, bitter melon is used to treat diabetes in Asia. It has twice as much potassium as bananas and is proven to increase the number of beta cells (which produce insulin) in the pancreas. It is high in iron and has twice the beta-carotene of broccoli and twice the calcium of spinach. It is bitter in taste and cooling to the body, but is too cooling and bitter for winter.

Best season: spring, summer
Carb predominant
Fat low
Protein low

BLACKBERRIES, RASPBERRIES

Native to Europe, these berries are harvested in late spring and early summer, from April through July, but are out of season in the winter and too cool for most winter climates. They are sweet, sour, and astringent and help to cool the body down and to treat diarrhea, a classic summer condition in which the stool is liquefied by excess heat. Blackberries and raspberries are very alkaline, high in iron, and are the best blood builders, although they can have a constipating quality.

Best season: summer
Protein 5.4 g
Fat 3.6–6 g
Carb 59.9 g

BLACK GRAM BEANS (SEE LEGUMES)

BLUEBERRIES

Native to North America, blueberries are harvested from May through August and are both sweet and astringent. Traditionally known to help strengthen the pancreas and stabilize blood sugar levels, blueberries serve to offset the high energy demands and high sugar content of the summer fruit harvest. They are not as cooling as blackberries or raspberries and are okay in winter. Recent studies have found blueberries to be a very powerful antioxidant.

Best season: spring, summer
Protein 2.9 g
Fat 2.1 g
Carb 63.8 g

BROCCOLI

Harvested in the summer and sometimes in the spring, broccoli is sweet, astringent, and cool. It is good both in spring and summer but is too light, dry, and gas producing (due to its sulfur content) for winter, unless well cooked with oil or ghee. (Steamed and then sautéed in olive oil and garlic, broccoli is especially delicious.) It is a good blood and liver cleanser with anti-cancer properties, and is high in vitamins A and C.

Best season: summer
Protein 9.1 g
Fat .6 g
Carb 15.2 g

BRUSSELS SPROUTS

More astringent and with a higher sulfur content than broccoli, Brussels sprouts are harvested much later, from November to December. They are too hot and pungent for summer, but if well cooked provide a high protein source in the winter. Brussels sprouts are best if cooked or baked in a casserole, as they are heavy, somewhat hard to digest, and gas producing. With many concentrated nutrients, these unpopular vegetables help slow the thyroid for the long, less active winter months. Because they are so concentrated and hardy, they easily store into spring, when they make a good liver cleanser and nutrient source with anti-cancer properties.

Best season: winter, spring
Protein 29 g
Fat 2.3 g
Carb 40.8 g

BUCKWHEAT

Originally from China with roots in Russia (as kasha), buckwheat is a heating and drying grain with astringent and pungent properties. A bit too hot for summer, it is all right in winter if not eaten in excess. It is a great grain antidote for spring and a perfect wheat alternative.

Best season: spring
Protein 24 g
Fat 3 g
Carb 173 g
(8 oz.)

BUTTER

As with most dairy products, butter is fine in winter and summer and should be reduced in the spring. For some it is easy to avoid dairy products, but for most Americans this is a difficult task. One tip to make it easier is to eat butter only at breakfast and lunch and avoid it at night. The body digests all food better at midday, and a heavy food like butter is less aggravating if avoided at night. See ghee for a natural butter substitute; natural margarine and soy margarines are also acceptable in moderation during the spring.

Best season: winter
Protein 9 g
Fat 11 g
Carb 9 g
(14 g)

BUTTERMILK

Anytime dairy is cultured, it will change from a cooling food that is acceptable in the summer to a heating food to be avoided in the summer. These foods are always acceptable in small amounts around meals as their heating effect will stimulate digestive strength. Cultured dairy products are still best in the winter, however, like all dairy. These include kefir, sour cream, and yogurt.

Best season: winter
Protein 9 g
Fat 19 g
Carb 12 g
(Based on 1 cup whole yogurt)

CABBAGE

Loaded with minerals, particularly calcium, and high in vitamins C and A, cabbage is usually harvested in the spring. It has been used traditionally for skin conditions, ulcers, constipation, and circulatory disorders.

Best season: spring, summer
Protein 4.6 g
Fat .7 g
Carb 17.5 g

CARROTS

Sweet, slightly pungent, warm, and harvested in the fall, carrots are especially beneficial in winter and spring and too heating for summer if eaten

242 THE 3-SEASON DIET

in excess. They are high in vitamin A and are good for the eyes, and their high calcium content makes them great for bones, muscles, and teeth. They increase the flow of blood and lymph and reduce swelling, inflammations, and liver conditions.

Best season: winter, spring
Protein 4.8 g
Fat 1.2 g
Carb 37.2

CAULIFLOWER

Part of the cabbage family along with broccoli, Brussels sprouts, and kale, cauliflower is astringent, sweet, and cool. It is harvested in the spring and summer, and some varieties in the winter. Its high sulfur and phosphorus content makes it gas forming, but cooking it well with oil, fennel, cumin, and hing renders it more digestible in winter. Wind is high in winter, so if you want to eat a wind-producing food you must cook and spice it appropriately.

Best season: spring, summer
Protein 4.9 g
Fat .4 g
Carb 19 g

CELERY

Harvested in the spring and summer, celery is a highly alkaline food good for neutralizing acids, which are high after a long winter of nuts and grains. It mixes well with almost anything and juices very readily. Celery has a high mineral content, rich in sodium, potassium, and sulfur. With an astringent, sweet, and slightly salty taste, it is a well-known diuretic and blood purifier as well as a tonic for the nervous system and good for blood pressure. It can be eaten raw in the spring or summer and can be cooked into soups and stews in the winter.

Best season: spring, summer
Protein 1.8 g
Fat 3.18 g
Carb 51.4 g

CHEESES

Sweet and somewhat cooling, most cheeses are best in the winter as they are high in protein and fat and so counteract dryness. They are all right in moderation in the summer, but the saltier and harder cheeses will be more heating then. Softer cheeses like cream cheese and cottage cheese are less likely to overheat the body. Nonetheless, summer types should avoid cheese in the summer, and spring types especially should avoid them in spring, since cheese will increase mucus production. Cottage cheese is the best cheese in the summer and is acceptable in moderation in spring if eaten at midday.

Best season: winter

Protein 8 g

Fat 5 g

Carb 1 g

(1 oz. whole-milk mozzarella; other cheeses vary greatly in fat content.)

CHERRIES

Typically harvested in June and July, cherries are one of the first fruits of the summer season. When ripe and sweet off the tree, they help to cool the body for the coming heat. Blood builders with a very high iron and carbohydrate content, cherries help give the body strength and energy for the long days and short nights of summer. Their heavy iron content and sweet taste make them a bit too heavy for the spring, but cherries are fine in the winter if fully ripened.

Best season: early summer

Protein 5.3 g

Fat 1.2 g

Carb 71 g

CHICKEN (TURKEY)

Lighter than beef, poultry is sweet, warm, and still primarily a winter food. It has a much higher carbohydrate content than beef as well, so it can be eaten in moderation (and preferably at the noon meal) in the spring and summer. Winter types typically need more meat all year long, and poultry is a good alternative to red meat. Because turkey is somewhat heavier than chicken, summer types should eat it in moderation in the summer, or at least at the midday meal rather than at night. The overuse of hormones and pesticides in feed makes it well worth spending a few cents a pound extra to buy free-range, natural poultry whenever possible.

Best Season: winter
Protein 18 g
Fat 13 g
Carb 0 g
(1 cutlet)

CHICORY

Related to endive, chicory is a leafy green whose root and greens can both be eaten, although most use just the green tops. It is a high-alkaline spring food rich in vitamin C, a blood and liver cleanser, and should be abundant in the markets in the spring.

Best season: spring
Protein 6.7 g
Fat 1.1 g
Carb 14.1 g

CHILIES (HOT PEPPERS)

Harvested in the late spring and summer, the many varieties of chilies are best used as a medicine to help digest heavy foods. Too many in summer can overheat the body. Tropical cultures often overuse this food as a digestive agent and in an attempt to ward off infections and food pathogens, such as parasites and amoebas that flourish in the tropics. Tropical climates are wet, and the pepper helps combat the humid, mucus-producing environment. Chilies are best used dried for spicing heavy winter foods, or in the spring to break up excess mucus production. They are also great medicine for colds, asthma, and other respiratory conditions.

Best season: winter, spring
Protein 2.1 g
Fat .5 g
Carb 10.7 g
(1 cup)

CILANTRO (CORIANDER)

Those who don't tolerate heat must take notice of cilantro in the summer, as it is one of the most cooling foods on earth. Good for food, skin, and seasonal allergies, it purifies the blood, bile, and kidneys. If taken with chilies in the summer (it is present in most Mexican and many Indian dishes) it will neutralize the heating effects of the chilies and curries. Cilantro, also called coriander, is a good spring cleanser and can be taken in smaller amounts in winter.

Best season: summer
Protein .2 g
Fat .3 g
Carb 1 g
(1 tsp.)

COCONUTS

In the south of India, which the natives say was the birthplace of the first coconut tree, they call it the tree of life–given to them by God to feed, house, dress, and cure them. Coconut is basically cooling, as it is a staple in many tropical climates. According to local people, its milk is akin to mother's milk and is considered a complete protein. This fruit is harvested all year long, but the ripe nut with the most white coconut meat is available mostly in the winter, as it is 70 percent fat and a perfect winter antidote for the tropics. The green coconut milk is said to be a medicine for the skin with a very cooling effect.

Best season: green coconut—summer
ripe coconut—summer, winter
Protein: 15.9 g
Fat 160.1 g
Carb 42.6 g

COLLARD GREENS (SEE KALE)

CORN

The origins of corn are still unknown. Some of the oldest records show maize being grown in ancient India some 5,000 years ago. Traditionally it was more abundant in tropical climates than in the northern climates where it is now raised. Although the U.S. "corn belt" comprises Iowa and Illinois, for instance, corn in this hemisphere is actually indigenous to Mexico, where it was originally harvested before the late winter monsoons, to be eaten in the wettest time of year there. It made perfect sense to harvest the driest grain before the wettest time of year. Cornmeal is a very dry and heating grain as well, perfect as an antidote for spring's moisture. In the North corn was harvested in the fall and ground into cornmeal to be eaten as a warming grain for the winter and, if supplies lasted, as a dry grain for the spring. In the South grits are still a common hot cereal taken mostly for its warming effect in the winter and the wet spring. Fresh corn will heat up the body only if eaten in excess, so sweet fresh corn is still an appropriate end-of-summer food here in America.

Best season: spring
Protein 11.9 g
Fat 3.9 g
Carb 66.9 g

CRANBERRIES

One of the last berries harvested before winter, the cranberry is a transitional food bridging the gap between summer and winter. The berries are astringent, sour, and sweet, and they offer us the last chance to cool the blood and remove the excess heat from the long, hot summer. They are also an acid food, unlike most summer fruits and veggies, which are alkaline. The cooling property combined with its acid nature (which is more appropriately a winter quality) make cranberries a great transition food to start the rebuilding process of winter. The cranberry is much like the cherry, which is the first summer-harvested fruit and helps to make the transition from spring to summer.

Best season: late summer
Protein 1.8 g
Fat 3.18 g
Carb 51.4

CUCUMBERS

Sweet, cooling, astringent, the cuke is a classic summer balancing food whose refrigerant and diuretic properties help the body stay cool in the heat. It cools the blood—hence, "as cool as a cucumber." Cukes are a digestive aid and when combined with yogurt (which is heating) make a perfectly balanced food (as in the Indian dish known as *raita*).

Best season: summer
Protein 2.2 g
Fat .3 g
Carb 8.6 g

DANDELIONS

A member of the sunflower family harvested in the spring and throughout the summer, the dandelion is high in vitamin A and potassium. It is best known as a liver cleanser and bile-flow stimulator. This is a useful food in spring, when the liver is working hard to detoxify the deep tissues and fat cells. Deer instinctively chew on the surface rhizomes and leaves of the dandelion, both of which are bitter and support the liver's seasonal cleansing process. For a spring treat, try dandelion tea: Boil dandelion leaves in water, add a pinch of salt, and drink throughout the day. The bitter taste actually grows on you!

Best season: spring and summer
Protein 12.3 g
Fat 3.2 g
Carb 49 g

DATES

Harvested in the fall, dates are sweet and heavy and are a perfect antidote to winter's cold, drying winds. Dates are considered a rejuvenative, a tonic, an aphrodisiac, and a great source of copper, which is necessary for iron absorption. These building qualities are especially important in the winter when the body is trying to store protein, fat, minerals, and vitamins. With milk, dates are good for ulcers and for children with weak stomachs. They are also used as a reproductive tonic and lung conditioner.

Best season: winter
Protein 8.7 g
Fat 2.4 g
Carb 297 g

DUCK

Harder to digest than chicken or turkey but still easier than beef.

Best season: winter
Protein 28 g
Fat 8 g
Carb 9 g
(3 oz. portion)

EGGPLANT

Eggplant is generally cooling and best in the summer. Depending on the location, however, it can be harvested all year long. If well cooked in oil or baked with appropriate winter spices (pepper, garlic, onions), it is fine in winter but should be avoided in spring owing to its high water content. Because it is a nightshade, eggplant may aggravate arthritis and allergies. It is generally advised to take this food in moderation in any season.

Best season: summer
Protein 4.3 g
Fat .8 g
Carb 21.7 g

EGGS

A better choice than meats for a high-quality complete protein, eggs are sweet and warm and, like meats, are best taken in the winter. In spring and summer they can be eaten in moderation at breakfast or a midday meal. Egg whites are cooling and egg yolks are heating, although I do not recommend separating the two.

Best season: winter
Protein 6 g
Fat 5.5 g
Carb .6 g

FENNEL

Fennel is a sweet and warm vegetable resembling celery, but with the flavor of anise. Its peak season is from September to February but it is good in all seasons. It is used traditionally as a digestive agent and can be eaten raw or cooked.

Best season: all
Protein: 1.1 g
Fat: .2 g
Carb: 6.3 g
(1 cup)

FIGS

With their peak harvest occurring in the fall, figs are a transitional food from summer to winter. Their cooling properties make them a good summer antidote and a sweet, heavy, and nutritive balance for winter's cold and dryness. When dried they are acceptable in spring. Figs are also demulcent and laxative and are great liver and kidney tonics. The heat of summer and dryness of winter can cause constipation and dryness, and the transition from summer to winter can put excess stress on the liver and kidneys, making figs a perfect choice.

Best season: end of summer, winter
Protein 6 g
Fat 2 g
Carb 89 g

FRESHWATER FISH

Good in all seasons, although all meats and fish are best consumed in winter. Fish are high in omega 3 fatty acids, which help lower cholesterol and triglycerides. Think of Eskimos eating fish in Alaska—the high fatty acid content insulates them for the long winter months. Unlike saltwater fish that heat the body owing to their salt content, freshwater fish are without salt so they cool the body for summer, and they do not hold on to water, so are good in spring as well. Because of contamination of water sources with pollutants, it is best to buy all fish from a fish farm unless you know the source.

Best season: all
Protein 21 g

Fat 6 g
Carb 9 g

GARLIC

Harvested in the spring and fall, garlic is best during those seasons. Its hot and pungent nature make it a bit hot for summer, but it provokes a stimulating and cleansing response in the body in the spring and fall (when most roots are harvested). Some cultures treat garlic as a medicine rather than a food and it should not be overused. Taking it every day as a preventative for blood pressure problems or colds for months on end is not unlike how we overuse antibiotics, which have become ineffective against many of the bacteria they were designed to kill. Use garlic both as a food in the winter and spring and moderately in the summer to spice your food; put it in your cupboard to be used as a medicine against a cold when it comes. With antibiotics rendered increasingly less effective, you may need an herb like garlic that will give clinical antibiotic results at your disposal. It is good for infections, edema, depression, fatigue, parasites, yeast infections, and numerous other conditions.

Best season: spring, winter
Protein 24 g
Fat 1 g
Carb 123 g

GHEE

Ghee, also known as clarified butter, is raw butter with the heavy milk solids skimmed off during boiling. The result is a lighter butter that can be used as a spread, for cooking, and even as a topical medicine for burns or skin irritations. As a butter substitute, it is acceptable in winter, summer, and, if eaten in moderation, spring as well. Remember that spring is a low-fat time of year, so don't overdo it. For sleep disorders, ghee can be rubbed on the feet and head before bedtime, as it calms the nervous system.

Best season: winter, summer
Protein 9 g
Fat 14 g
Carb 9 g
(1 tbs.)

GINGER

Known as the universal spice, ginger can be taken in all seasons, but may increase heat in the summer if used in excess. It is primarily a digestive and a diaphoretic used to increase sweating during a cold or flu. Ginger in tea or carbonated drinks is great for nausea, constipation, and diarrhea. The powder is hotter than the fresh root, and both are often mixed with honey and then used as a medicine. The powder can be mixed into a paste with water for headaches and joint pain.

Best season: spring, winter

Protein .4 g

Fat .3 g

Carb 3 g

GRAPEFRUIT

Depending on the location, grapefruit can be available all year long, although they are primarily in season from January to May, making them a great transition fruit from winter to spring. Sour, sweet, and heavy due to their high water content, grapefruit are the perfect antidote for winter. In the spring they have a unique ability to break up mucus that is often a problem in "allergy season." Because of the sour taste they can be too heating in the summer, particularly for summer types. A grapefruit in the morning with honey is a fine way to break up any congestion accumulated during the night. Rich in vitamin C, the seed has become a popular antioxidant and natural antibiotic. Grapefruit's ability to break up mucus has given it a reputation for being a weight-loss agent, although this is limited at best.

Best season: winter

Protein 2 g

Fat 1 g

Carb 39 g

GRAPES

Harvested from July through March, with their peak between August and November in the United States, grapes are available year round from all over the world. They are sweet, cooling, and heavy, making them good for the summer and winter, but too heavy for spring. Their high magnesium content helps to maintain good elimination, and they are natural cleansers for the kidney and bladder. The seed is a powerful antioxidant. In the spring, dried grapes or raisins are best.

Best season: late summer, winter
Protein 4 g
Fat 2 g
Carb 74 g

GUAVA

High in vitamin C, guava is a tropical fruit with primarily cooling properties. It is good in the summer but also in the winter because of the heavy and sweet nature of its nectar. It is excellent for the lymphatic and skeletal systems.

Best season: summer
Protein 4 g
Fat 3 g
Carb 66 g

ICE CREAM

Like most dairy products, ice cream is cooling and so is best in summer. It should be avoided in winter and especially in spring (it significantly increases mucus production), and should not be eaten at night.

Best season: summer
Protein 22 g
Fat 18 g
Carb 5 g
(Häagen-Dazs, chocolate, ½ cup)

JICAMA

Sometimes called yam bean or Mexican turnip, jicama is a legume that is grown for its large tuberous root, which can be eaten raw or cooked. It is predominately a starch, harvested before the frost, and is cooling for the accumulated heat at the end of summer. It is also an astringent vegetable, making it good in spring. Jicama can be stored and cooked for winter much like a white potato.

Best season: summer (raw), winter (cooked)
Carb predominately starch

KALE (COLLARD GREENS, SWISS CHARD)

Like other cabbage family vegetables, kale is astringent and primarily a blood purifier. It is available in the spring, when it helps the liver cleanse the blood, and in summer, when it acts as a natural cooling agent to combat accumulated heat. In the winter if cooked with oil or ghee, kale can be eaten in moderation. There are many indigenous varieties of kale, including red, green, and purple, all with similar properties. Collard greens have an extremely high calcium content–357 mg/cup. They are also high in Vitamins A and C. Swiss chard, unlike kale, will heat up the body if eaten in excess.

Best season: spring, summer
Protein 11 g
Fat 2 g
Carb 21 g

LAMB

Too heavy for spring and too heating for summer, lamb is best eaten in winter, like all red meat.

Best season: winter
Protein 24 g
Fat 6 g
Carb 9 g
(3 oz.)

LEEKS (SEE ONIONS)

LEGUMES

Generally, legumes are sweet and astringent. They tend to be light and gas producing, so most should be avoided in the winter. They have a hard shell that allows them to be safely stored during the winter months to be eaten in spring and summer. In nature, legumes lie on the ground all winter and sprout in the spring. Animals eat these sprouts faster than they can grow—and so should we in the spring. In the winter legumes are acidic in nature, but in the spring they become alkaline when they sprout. When cooked with winter spices like cumin, hing, fennel, salt, onions, and pepper, legumes are more easily digested (particularly in the winter). Certain legumes stand alone from the rest and are all right to eat in winter, as they do not have gas-producing properties: mung beans—especially split yellow mung beans—and tofu (see Soybeans, Tofu).

Best season: spring, summer
See individual beans for Protein, Fat, and Carb content.

LEMONS

Traditionally lemons were harvested in the winter, although they are now available all year long. Their sour taste has a heating effect that acts as an antidote to the cold of winter. They are also available in the spring and help to break up the mucus generated by dampness. With honey, lemon juice is a good expectorant and digestive. Its heating properties, much like those of hot peppers, are available as a digestive medicine much of the year. Lemonade, the classic summer drink, is cooling mostly because of the sweeteners and water content. The lemon has an initial refrigerant or cooling property followed by an internal heating property that supports digestion because of its sour taste, without overheating the stomach. This is also why it has been successful with heartburn.

Best season: winter
Protein 3 g
Fat 1 g
Carb 48 g

LENTILS

Harvested in the fall, lentils are a legume or bean, which means they produce gas. If eaten in the winter, they are a protein source as rich as many meats, but they need to be soaked and cooked for an extended time to reduce their gas-producing properties. The hard shell of a lentil or any bean makes it safe to store for the winter and a great food for spring. In nature they would lie dormant on the ground all winter and sprout naturally in the spring. The animals feast on them during the spring and so should we. (Beans turn from an acid, high-protein, building food in the winter to a high-alkaline, cleansing food in the spring.)

Best season: spring (as bean or sprouted)
Protein 112 g
Fat 5 g
Carb 272 g

LETTUCE

The many varieties of lettuce are all cooling and slightly astringent, making them good in the spring and summer. They have typically diuretic properties and are blood and lymph purifiers. The greener the leaf, as in romaine or greenleaf lettuce, for example, the more iron and other minerals are present, along with vitamins A and C. The classic head lettuce sold in America as iceberg, recognizable by its tightly packed leaves, is a hybrid developed in the 16th century. Although it tastes good, it offers minimal nutrition beyond fiber and alkaline properties. Originally lettuce had long stems with large leaves looking more like leafy greens.

Best season: spring, summer
Protein 4 g
Fat 1 g
Carb .5 g

LIMA BEANS

Very astringent and sweet, limas are good in the spring and summer. In the winter they are too gas provoking. Although harvested in the fall in America, they originated in Guatemala, where the winters are mild and a gas-producing or winter-aggravating bean would not matter. Its anti-mucus and cooling properties were necessary in the humid tropics.

Best season: spring
Protein 14 g
Fat 2 g
Carb 43 g

LIMES

Native to southeastern Asia, the lime is mainly harvested in the winter. Much like the lemon, with which it is often paired, it is best in winter and somewhat good in spring. It is slightly more cooling than the lemon in the summer. Limes are high in vitamins C, B$_1$, and potassium and are also a great alkalizer for the body and a coolant for the nervous system. They are useful against heatstroke, fevers, and heart palpitations, and are good for digestive disorders.

Best season: winter

Protein 3 g

Fat 1 g

Carb 42 g

MANGOES

Native to India but now grown throughout the Western tropics from Haiti to Ecuador, the mango is a sweet, sour, and slightly warm fruit. Harvested from May through September, it is highly nutritious with cooling properties for the summer when the fruit is totally ripe. It is also sweet and sour, making it a perfect winter antidote, but is slightly heavy for spring. All aspects of the mango have traditionally been used as medicine. The skin is very astringent and taken for loose bowels, while the fruit is a tonic for the nervous system. Unripe mangoes are pickled and used to stimulate digestion.

Best season: summer, winter

Protein 2 g

Fat 1 g

Carb 52 g

MELONS

Originated in Asia, New Guinea, and India, melons provide great cooling relief for a tropical climate and for the summer months above and below the equator. They are great in the summer, but too heavy for the spring and too cooling for winter. In the tropics, however, they are appropriate all year long. Melons are loaded with distilled water, minerals, and vitamins A, B, and C and typically provide end-of-summer nutritional support and cooling relief.

Best season: summer

Protein 1 g

Fat .5 g
Carb 14 g

MILK

Milk is sweet, cool, and heavy, good in summer, fine in winter if not drunk cold and in excess. In the spring, milk should generally be avoided or at least be drunk in its low-fat version as it is too mucus producing. It is a rejuvenative and a tonic for the nervous and reproductive systems. Milk has gotten a bad reputation lately because of the growth hormones and antibiotics given to cows in the West. These adulterations added to the pasteurization and homogenization processes render most store-bought milk chemically quite different from what nature intended the cow to feed her calves. Many ethnic groups do not have the enzymes to break milk down and should avoid it altogether. Others are sensitive to store-bought milk, which is difficult to digest primarily because of the homogenization process.

Best season: summer
Protein 11 g
Fat 8 g
Carb 8 g
(1 cup whole milk)

MILLET

A high-protein wheat alternative excellent in spring, millet has a heating energy that can irritate summer types in the long days of August and should be reduced. In the winter, millet will heat up the body against the cold, but should not to be eaten in excess because of its dry nature.

Best season: spring
Protein 3 g
Fat .5 g
Carb 19 g
(1 cup)

MOLASSES

What we call molasses is simply pure sugar cane juice of varying levels of extraction. The level of lowest quality but greatest taste appeal is blackstrap. Molasses is sweet and cooling, but due to its unrefined state is too heavy in summer. It is high in iron and traditionally used as a tonic for the heart, blood, and muscles.

Best season: winter, spring
Protein 0
Fat 0
Carb 13 g
(1 tbs)

MUNG BEANS

Mungs are one of the few beans that balance the effects of all three seasons. They are particularly useful in the summer, as they will cool the body and supply high amounts of protein. Cooked with rice into a soup, they make a tonic for children, postpartum women, and convalescence or any debilitated condition. Medicines were traditionally cooked into this soup to make them more easily digested. Mung beans are acid in nature but will not heat the body like most acid foods. Sprouted in the spring and summer, they become alkaline and rich in minerals and chlorophyll needed to clean and cool the blood. Unlike most beans, mungs produce little gas and are actually beneficial in the winter, making it the winter bean of choice.

Best season: all, winter
Protein 15 g
Fat trace
Carb 38 g
(1 cup)

MUSHROOMS

Harvested in wet, moist regions usually in the spring, when the earth is saturated with water. The sweet, astringent, and pungent nature of mushrooms makes for a perfect spring antidote. They move excess fluid out of the body and they have anti-tumor and anti-cancer properties. Mushrooms are a rare source of germanium and B vitamins, which help the adrenals fight stress and strengthen the nervous system. They are also available in the summer but should be avoided in winter, as they are too astringent and dry.

Best season: spring
Protein 12 g
Fat 1 g
Carb 19 g

MUSTARD GREENS

Native to northwest India, mustard greens have long provided a leafy green that is good in the winter and spring and slightly heating in the summer, and in northern India this heating property is welcome. The greens as well as their seeds are used there as expectorants to break up congestion during winter- and springtime colds. In America we can use mustard greens to help with allergies and congestion in winter and spring, and as a medicinal food in the summer, while most other leafy greens will provide the needed summer cooling influence.

Best season: spring
Protein 19 g
Fat 1 g
Carb 18 g

NECTARINES (SEE PEACHES)

Nectarines are similar to peaches, although their skin is less aggravating to heat-sensitive types. They are slightly easier on summer types in the hot summer months. As with peaches, it's best to eat them only when they are totally ripe.

NUTS

Harvested in the late summer to be eaten in the winter, nuts are a high-protein, high-fat food that in America are typically eaten least when they are most needed—in the winter. They are strengthening, tonic, rejuvenative, and good for the reproductive and nervous systems. In spring and summer they should be eaten in moderation or soaked in water overnight to enhance digestibility. Exceptions to this rule include coconuts, macadamia nuts, and lotus seed, which are cooling in summer. Flax, piñons, (pine nuts), and pumpkin seeds are warm and dry and good in the spring and winter.

Best season: winter
Protein 5.3 g
Fat 15.4 g
Carb 5.5 g
(1 oz. almonds)

OATS

Heavy, cool, and sweet, oats are a great tonic for the nervous system. Cooked, they are heavy and nutritious for winter and slightly cooling for summer. In the spring they should be eaten dry or in moderation. Oats are naturally demulcent and great for chronic constipation.

Best season: winter
Protein 5 g
Fat 2.5 g
Carb 23 g
(1 cup)

OCEAN FISH

Sweet and salty, saltwater fish like tuna and halibut are generally good in the winter but because of the salt are too heating for summer and hold on to too much water for spring. In moderation, however, they will not overheat the body in the summer, although summer types should take more caution. In the spring if eaten in moderation, they can serve as a meat alternative, but spring types should take more caution. Lighter fish like sole are easier to digest in all seasons.

Best season: winter
Protein 31 g
Fat 8.8 g
Carb 0 g
(1 halibut fillet—6 oz.)

OILS

Derived from nuts, beans, seeds, oily vegetables, and animal fats, oils are generally sweet, heavy, and warming. Vegetable oils are manufactured after the plants are fully ripe and harvested, typically in the fall to be eaten in the winter. The oil derived from the process (usually cold pressing) acts as a perfect winter antidote as it insulates the body from the cold, dry winter. In Scandinavian countries, people start taking cod liver oil or castor oil in the fall and continue throughout the winter to supplement Vitamin D and prevent common colds. Alaskans consume large amounts of fish oils for the same reason. In Mexico, where the winters are less severe, nature provides natural fruit oils from coconuts and avocados. In the contiguous United States we get our oils from nuts, grains, and meats. Depending on your geographical needs, nature will always harvest the perfect insulator for winter.

Best season: winter
Protein 0 g
Fat 220 g
Carb 0 g
(1 cup olive oil)

OKRA

Okra, a tropical vegetable native to Africa, is sweet and cooling and a good summer heat antidote. If cooked well it can also be a good winter vegetable. It has a high amount of vegetable mucin, a viscid substance that acts as a demulcent and a lubricant for irritated intestinal membranes. The same lubricating properties that help to relieve inflammatory conditions such as ulcers, diarrhea, dysentery, and joint pain will, however, increase mucus production in the spring and should be reduced at that time.

Best season: summer
Protein 9 g
Fat 1 g
Carb 39 g

ONIONS

Thought to have originated in Asia, onions are harvested in the spring in warm climates and in the fall in cold climates. They are best eaten in spring and winter and are too spicy or pungent for the summer. When well cooked, they lose their spiciness and are acceptable in summer in moderation, except for summer types. They are best in winter when cooked, but raw they are fine in spring. Leeks are like onions but have milder properties. They are useful for colds, general debility, and nervous system disorders. If you are sensitive to onions, eat them with parsley to counter the sulfurous effect in the intestinal tract.

Best season: spring
Protein 6 g
Fat .5 g
Carb 36 g

ORANGES

Harvested in the winter, oranges are sweet and sour and heavy, making them a perfect winter-balancing food. They are cooling except for the sour varieties, which will heat up the body. But they are too heavy for spring and should be avoided. Conversely, sour varieties are all right as a medicinal food in spring because they break up mucus in the respiratory tract. They are high in vitamin C, good for elimination and colds.

Best season: winter
Protein 3 g
Fat 1 g
Carb 36 g

PAPAYAS

Native to Central America, papayas are basically sweet, heavy, and slightly warm and are typically harvested all year long. Their abundance of natural digestive enzymes makes them ideal in winter, when they will keep the digestive furnace burning. Indeed, they can be eaten any time of year either alone or with other foods to enhance digestibility. Papayas balance blood sugar levels, are good for menstrual regularity, and are antiparasitic. In the summer they heat the body as it heats the digestion up, so if eaten in the summer they work best in a fruit salad with other cooling fruits to enhance digestibility. In the spring they can be eaten in moderation only, because they add heaviness to the season.

Best season: winter
Protein 2 g
Fat .5 g
Carb 39 g

PARSLEY

Native to southern Europe, parsley grown in warm southern climates is harvested all year long except for midsummer, when it is too hot. In extremely hot climates, parsley can overheat the body if eaten in excess. In the north it is available from early spring until late autumn and is one of the greens that can be eaten all year long, even in winter, as it does have warming properties. It is a very high-alkaline and blood-purifying food with natural diuretic properties that are much needed in the spring, when parsley is primarily harvested. Just as the earth holds on to more water in the spring, so does the body hold on to more fluid in an attempt to flush toxins from the deep tissues. Greens like parsley, with natural diuretic properties, are nature's seasonal response to the body's tendency to hold on to more water at this time of year.

Best season: spring
Protein 16 g
Fat 3 g
Carb 39 g

PEAS

Thought to have originated in central Europe or central Asia, peas are harvested from March through July. They are rich in chlorophyll and alkaline properties and so are perfect to help prepare the body for summer. Their high chlorophyll content acts as a fertilizer in the intestines, promoting the growth of good bacteria. Without an abundance of chlorophyll-rich foods in the spring, bad bacteria and yeast can flourish in the gut. Peas are high in vitamins A, C, and B_1 and minerals such as iron and calcium. They are primarily a springtime food with cooling properties that make them helpful in summer as well. They are mostly sweet and astringent and are gas producing in winter when eaten raw, dried, or split. (Split pea soup is a good summer recipe for loosening the bowels.) Snow peas are somewhat more cooling than green peas and so are good in both spring and summer.

Best season: spring
Protein 14 g
Fat 19 g
Carb 36 g

PEANUTS

Classified as an oily legume rather than a true nut, the peanut does act more like a nut than a bean in terms of its effect on the body. It is oily, heavy, sweet, and warm and a natural source of protein, making it a very good winter food. It is too heavy for the spring and too heating for summer, although in moderation it is fine.

Best season: winter

Protein 19 g

Fat 36 g

Carb 14 g

(½ cup, roasted)

PEACHES

Probably of Chinese origin, peaches are sweet, slightly sour, and cool. The peak harvest for peaches is July and August. As they are harvested at the end of summer, they are appropriately cooling as long as they are totally ripe. When fully tree ripe, peaches are soothing for ulcers, colitis, and inflammatory conditions, particularly in the digestive system. Most store-bought peaches are more sour than sweet and will tend to heat the body rather than cool it. When peaches are tree ripe they are extremely sweet, juicy, and cooling. The skin is the part that is most heating and irritating, so if you are sensitive to peaches, try removing it. Because of their heavy and sweet quality, peaches are also fine to eat right up to and into the winter months. They have demulcent and laxative properties, which help the body cope with the onset of winter's dryness.

Best season: summer into winter

Protein 2 g

Fat .5 g

Carb 38 g

PEARS

Native to western Europe, the pear is most abundant at the end of the summer. Sweet and mildly astringent (some varieties can be heavy), it is a great cooling agent for the summer, and its heavy nature makes it more appropriate in the winter than its cousin the apple. Pears are also appropriate in the spring or winter depending on the variety and ripeness of the fruit. The crisp, more astringent varieties that are slightly less ripe are good in the spring, and the heavy, demulcent types that are more ripe are better in winter. High in vitamin C and iron, they are good for elimination, coughs, and breaking up mucus.

Best season: summer
Protein 2 g
Fat .5 g
Carb 38 g

PERSIMMONS

The peak season for harvesting persimmons is October through December. Native to China and Japan, persimmons are a sweet, soft, demulcent, and heavy fruit when ripe. As they are harvested in the early winter months, they combat the cold and dryness of winter if eaten ripe. In northern climates they are harvested in the late summer and act as good cooling fruits for the heat of summer. In this regard they are good medicine for heat-related conditions such as diarrhea and intestinal bleeding. In the winter they help soothe dry coughs.

Best season: summer, winter
Protein 3 g
Fat 2 g
Carb 73 g

PINEAPPLES

Native to tropical America, pineapples are generally available all year long depending on where they are harvested. Their peak season is June and July and when ripe and sweet they are very cooling for summer and summer types. Sour pineapples will heat up the body slightly. Sour varieties are especially good in the winter, however, when the sour heating effect is welcome. Pineapples are refrigerant, laxative, and digestive as they contain digestive enzymes. They are an especially good liver and blood cleanser. During the spring-summer transition, when the liver is working hard to cleanse the blood, pineapples will help the liver move the impurities more effectively.

Best season: summer
Protein 1 g

Fat .5 g
Carb 33 g

PLUMS, PRUNES

Probably a native of the West Indies, the prune is a variety of plum that can be dried without fermenting when the pit is not removed, although today the word is generally used to denote any dried plum. It is basically sweet and somewhat sour, laxative, heavy, and somewhat acid, whereas most fruits are alkaline. Plums are harvested in the summer and fall and are predominately cooling. In the spring they are hard to digest and too heavy. They make a better winter and summer food, as the slight sour taste warms against the winter and the sweet, ripe plums balance against the hot sun of summer.

Best season: summer
Protein 3 g
Fat 1 g
Carb 56 g

POMEGRANATES

Native to Persia, the pomegranate is one of the oldest fruits known to humanity. It is generally balancing for all seasons but is therapeutic in the summer because of its cooling nature. Harvested in late summer and fall, this fruit is timed to be eaten when the summer's heat is at its peak. After the trees turn bright red with accumulated heat of summer, the pomegranate is harvested to put out this fire. In warmer climates where the summer's heat lingers, it is harvested as late as December. Blessed with bile-, blood-, and liver-cleansing properties, it is also good for indigestion, hyperacidity, and diarrhea.

Best season: summer
Protein 1 g
Fat 1 g
Carb 42 g

PORK

Sweet and cool, pork is acceptable in the winter and summer but too heavy for spring.

Best season: winter, summer
Protein 19 g
Fat 25 g
Carb 0 g
(2.7 oz. pork chop)

POTATOES (WHITE)

Native to Central America, the potato is cool, sweet, and astringent. These tastes make the potato better in the spring and summer and not so good in the winter unless well cooked, mashed, or boiled in soup, and spiced with winter spices. Baked potatoes are excellent in the spring and in the summer and can be eaten in any fashion. Up to 60 percent of the potassium in potatoes is found just under the skin, so always try to eat them with the skin on; they are also fine raw, sliced thin on salads, or lightly cooked. High in vitamin C, the potato is a complete food and generally balances all seasons except winter in excess. There have been documented reports of people living on only potatoes for up to three years. As an indigenous tropical vegetable, it provides more cooling properties for warm climates than heating properties for cold climates.

Best season: summer, spring
Protein 7.5 g
Fat .5 g
Carb 7 g

PUMPKINS

Harvested during the late summer, pumpkins' peak is from October through December, depending on the climate. Pumpkin seeds are a perfect winter snack; they can be dried in the fall to be eaten all winter. Pumpkin meat is cooling, sweet, and heavy and is a great transition food from summer to winter. It is cooling for the end of summer and heavy and sweet for the dry winter months ahead. Pumpkin seeds are high in zinc, potassium, and sodium and are a well-known prostate remedy. With salt they are a good winter mineral source and snack.

Best season: early winter
Protein 4 g

Fat .5 g
Carb 21 g

QUINOA

Native to South America, quinoa (pronounced KEEN-wah) is sweet, astringent, and pungent and is a high-protein grain source for winter. A low-gluten grain, it is also beneficial in the spring. In summer, summer types should eat it in moderation.

Best season: winter, spring
Protein 5 g
Fat 2 g
Carb 28 g
(¼ cup flour)

RADISHES

Native to China and cultivated thousands of years ago in Egypt, radishes are typically harvested from April to July. They are pungent, astringent, light, and warm and are balancing for both spring and summer in moderation. They are too stimulating in the winter when the metabolism is lowered to promote rest during the short days and long nights. The pungent and stimulating nature of radishes is most useful in the spring when the body tends to hold on to more mucus and water. The radish is an expectorant and it can be used all year long as a medicine to help digest other foods.

Best season: spring
Protein 3 g
Fat .5 g
Carb 19 g

RICE

Rice is one of the more balanced foods. Brown rice is more nutritive than white rice, but it can be overheating if eaten in excess. White basmati rice is excellent for summer and winter but can be too sticky for springtime. In the spring and winter brown rice is best, as the husk increases digestive heat needed to breakup the mucus of spring and combat the cold of winter.

Best season: brown rice, winter; white rice, summer
Protein 3 g
Fat 9 g
Carb 38 g
(¼ cup basmati)

RYE

A sweet, astringent grain, rye is light enough to be eaten in the spring and cooling enough to be eaten in summer. It has strong diuretic properties and is good for removing water and mucus from spring types, particularly in the spring season.

Best season: spring
Protein 19 g
Fat 1.5 g
Carb 65 g
(1 cup flour)

SEAWEED

Salty, astringent, and cooling, seaweed is high in minerals and builds the blood. It is a well-known remedy for thyroid conditions, small tumors, and cysts and it helps to relieve swelling in the lymphatic system. It is generally good for all seasons but like all vegetables should be well cooked in winter. Because seaweed is high in chlorophyll, it helps the body fertilize good-bacteria growth in the intestines in the spring. Kelp, for example, is a rich source of vitamin B_{12} and should be consumed in large quantities when most other greens are consumed.

Best season: All
Protein 7.3 percent
Fat 1.5 percent
Fiber 46 percent

SHELLFISH

High in protein, clams, muscles, shrimp, lobster, and scallops are fine in the winter but are too heating and heavy for summer and spring.

Best season: winter
Protein 27 g

Fat 2 g
Carb 0 g
(1 cup lobster meat)

SNOW PEAS (SEE PEAS)

SOYBEANS, TOFU

Native to Europe, soybeans and tofu are sweet and astringent. The soybean is very high in protein and can be eaten in the winter when proteins are stored by the body, but it is excellent in the summer when the beans are harvested. It is one of the few beans that will not produce gas and aggravate winter health concerns, but it is heavy and slightly hard to digest for certain people. In the spring, soybeans should be reduced or eaten at midday, when a heavier food can be more easily digested. A natural source of phyto-estrogens that the body can convert into useful female hormones, soybeans and tofu are an essential piece of the nutritional puzzle for premenopausal women and vegetarians.

Best season: summer
Protein 158 g
Fat 89 g
Carb 152 g

SOY MILK

Because soybeans are better in the winter and summer, soy milk is best if taken during those seasons. It is less heavy than tofu and so is a good beverage in the spring.

Best season: all
Protein 3 g
Fat 2.5 g
Carb 10 g
(1 cup)

SPINACH

Spinach was introduced into China from the mountains of Nepal in the 7th century, but is believed to have originated in Persia, according to Bernard Jensen. Rich in vitamins and minerals, this tasty green is astringent, cool, and slightly pungent. As with most leafy greens, it is harvested in the spring and is loaded with chlorophyll and blood- and liver-cleansing properties. It's too cold a food for the winter unless well cooked; in summer it is generally good, but if not quite ripe and eaten in excess, it can heat up the body. Spinach salads in the spring and summer are perfect.

Best season: spring
Protein 19 g
Fat 1 g
Carb 15 g

STRAWBERRIES

This delicious berry is native to North and South America, but today's strawberry is a new fruit developed within the last 65 years through cross-pollination. It is a sweet, slightly sour, and astringent fruit, mainly harvested in summer (although some varieties can be picked as early as midspring), and it acts primarily as a cooling fruit. In the tropics where it originated, the strawberry was harvested earlier in the spring and acted as a blood purifier and cooling agent for a hot tropical environment. In moderation it can be eaten in spring and summer.

Best season: summer
Protein 4 g
Fat 3 g
Carb 35 g

SUMMER SQUASH, ACORN, AND OTHER VARIETIES (SEE ZUCCHINI)

SWEET POTATOES

Native to America, the sweet potato is a root vegetable, not a true tuber. Unlike the white potato, it is sweet and warm, heavier and more balancing for winter, but must be cooked well. It is so heavy it is sometimes hard to digest, particularly in the spring and summer. The yam is a different food, not widely grown in the U.S., but has similar properties to the sweet potato.

Best season: winter

Protein 6 g
Fat 2 g
Carb 97 g

SWISS CHARD (SEE KALE)

Best season: spring
Protein 6 g
Fat 1 g
Carb 17 g

TANGERINES (SEE ORANGES)

Not a hybrid, tangerines are from Tangiers or Morocco and are harvested in the winter like oranges.

Best season: winter
Protein 3 g
Fat 1 g
Carb 35 g

TOMATOES

Native to Peru and the Andes region of South America, the tomato is best in winter. It naturally heats the body, which was surely needed in the mountains of Peru. If eaten fresh and ripe off the vine and a sweet variety, it is all right in summer. Tomato sauces neutralized with sugar and spices are also okay in summer in moderation, but are still best in winter. You should reduce your tomato intake in the spring. Tomatoes are good medicine for the heart, circulation, cholesterol, cancer, and blood pressure, but if you have arthritis, avoid them.

Best season: winter
Protein 5 g
Fat 1 g
Carb 18 g

TURNIPS

Native to Siberia, the turnip is a root vegetable harvested in spring, like radishes and ginger. It is a powerful purifier of the blood, lymph, and liver. High in vitamin C, turnips help to break up mucus and congestion, particularly in the spring. They are also harvested in the fall, when the body again cleans the blood and lymph. The leafy green tops of turnips have the same properties as spinach.

Best season: spring
Protein 4 g
Fat 2 g
Carb 26 g

VEGETABLE OILS (SEE GROCERY LIST, APPENDIX 3)

VENISON
Primarily a winter food, venison (deer meat) is too warm and heavy for spring and summer.

Best season: winter
Protein 27 g
Fat 6.5 g
Carb 0 g
(3 oz.)

WATERCRESS
Native to Europe and America, watercress is a member of the mustard family. It is harvested in the spring and summer and is a powerful cooling food for summer, with blood-purifying properties for spring. It is a strong alkaline food that is effective in catarrh and glandular and toxic conditions.

Best season: spring, summer
Protein 8 g
Fat 1 g
Carb 15 g

WHEAT
A sweet, heavy, and slightly astringent grain with a high gluten content, wheat has gotten a bad name in America because of overconsumption. Like any other food, if you eat it in excess you will soon become oversensitive or allergic to it. Yet wheat is a superb winter grain because of its nutritive and strengthening properties. Substituting some of the other

grains, including rye, barley, or millet can help to desensitize the body to the high-gluten content of wheat. Eating wheat as crackers, nonyeasted bread, flat bread, or toasted bread helps to dry out its mucus-producing properties.

Best season: summer, winter
Protein 5 g
Fat .5 g
Carb 25 g
(¼ cup whole wheat flour)

WINTER SQUASH

Native to the Americas, the varieties of winter squashes are sweet, heavy, and warm compared to summer squash. They have a higher mineral and protein content and are harvested late in the summer to be eaten in the winter. They usually have demulcent properties to combat the dryness of winter and are good medicine for the dry, hacking coughs common in winter. They can also be eaten in the summer but are too heavy for spring.

Best season: winter
Protein 5 g
Fat 1 g
Carb 49 g

YOGURT (SEE BUTTERMILK)

ZUCCHINI

A sweet and cooling vegetable harvested in midsummer, zucchini is a blood purifier and a mild diuretic and refrigerant, making both the yellow and green varieties great anti-heat summer vegetables. In spring and winter they should be well cooked.

Best season: summer
Protein 5 g
Fat 1 g
Carb 19 g

REFERENCES FOR NUTRITIONAL FACTS

Jensen, Dr. Bernard. *Foods That Heal: A Guide to Understanding and Using the Healing Powers of Natural Foods.* Garden City Park, N.Y.: Avery Publishing Group, 1988.

Krause's Food, Nutrition, and Diet Therapy. L. Kathleen Mahan and Sylvia Escott-Stump, eds. Philadelphia, Pa.: W.B. Saunders Co., 1999

Kreutler, Patricia A. *Nutrition in Perspective.* Englewood Cliffs, N.J.: Prentice Hall, 1980.

Appendix 2

WHAT'S UNDER THE HOOD OF YOUR FOOD?

For years we have heard the debate about the value of organic food. Organics have traditionally cost more, sometimes twice as much as nonorganic produce, yet many of the chemical fertilizers and pesticides used in commercial farming are potential carcinogens that not only get into the foods we eat but have also contaminated our soil and water supplies, including our natural aquifers and oceans. Over the years, the most toxic chemicals have been restricted, but many remain on our foods and it is up to us to wash them off–if we can. The big business of growing food in such a surplus in the United States is no doubt having an impact on the environment. There are ways to grow foods while preserving the environment, but unless we are aware as consumers and make our demands heard, profit will dictate what we eat.

We are already exposed to so many environmental pollutants outside the foods we eat that we should at least eat foods that are as pure as possible, which is to say organically and naturally grown, free of irradiation and genetic engineering. When you eat out, you have no control over the chemicals you are ingesting, although some smart restaurants announce their use of organic produce on their menus. Mainstream grocery stores have begun carrying organic food for just pennies over the regular price. By buying these foods you are not only supporting the popularity of organic foods but, more important, you are supporting your local farmer and Mother Earth. In the years to come, your local farmer may be the only place you can get foods that are free of chemicals. Most local organic farmers do not use irradiation to extend shelf life, plant genetically engineered food, or irrigate crops with recycled sewage–even though the law says that such foods can be labeled organic. There are many planting techniques that mimic nature's balance on a farm so that insects do not devour all the corn or tomatoes. There are also certain natural pesticides–for example, neem, which is the leaf of a common tree in Asia now being used as a pesticide in Australia–that could have a great impact on reducing chemicals. Neem is banned in the United States as a pesticide but is approved as a food supplement.

I have included in this appendix a list of organic farmers in most areas of the country, along with numerous associations that could provide you with more information on the topic.

GENETIC ENGINEERING

A growing number of scientists and physicians are voicing concern over the possible health and environmental risks from the technology known as genetic engineering. For years the use of cross-pollination and hybridization techniques have transferred genes from one variety of corn to another. Nobody expressed concern because much the same thing already happens in nature at a somewhat slower speed. But genetic engineering is qualitatively different because it exchanges genes from one species to another. For example, many of the tomatoes on your grocery store shelves are genetically enhanced with genes from a flounder so that they will resist frosts. Did you know that? The FDA says that this kind of manipulation does not have to be labeled on the foods, and that even organic foods can be genetically altered in such a way.

Currently many such foods have made it to the marketplace without our knowledge, including soy, corn, squash, potatoes, tomatoes, and dairy products. They have all been altered to extend shelf life and resist insects, fungi, and viruses. Genetic engineers have attempted to improve on Mother Nature, but as you may have guessed by now, I am a big believer in the intelligence of nature and believe in a hands-off policy when it comes to trying to improve upon it. We have no clear way to know the long-term effects of genetically altered foods on us or the environment. Yet once they have been introduced, they will cross-pollinate with other species and there is no way to recall them as you would a faulty automobile or a defective lot of processed food.

One of the selling points of genetically engineered foods is that they are resistant to insects and do not require pesticides. This sounds great at first blush, but we are solving one problem only to create a host of others. If an insect that lived on corn as its major source of food forever now won't touch it because it doesn't recognize the corn as corn anymore, should *we* eat that corn? How will our bodies respond to it over time? And what happens to the insect who survived on corn, and the birds who fed their young with these insects, and so on down the road?

To do all this without the public's consent, or at least labeling requirements for such foods, seems more than reckless on the part of our government.

Even more astonishing to me is the creation of the new "terminator" technology, which alters a plant's genetic makeup to ensure that the plant will not go to seed. The farmer will be forced to buy seeds each year from one manufacturer, and, of course, these seeds will all be genetically altered in any way the manufacturer chooses with what amounts to no government restrictions. Soon good seeds that are pure, organic, and genetically intact are going to be in great demand. I have included in this appendix all the suppliers of organic and heirloom seeds, some of which date back to the 1800s, before anyone even began hybridizing many of these plants. If you've ever seen or tasted some of the wonderful tomatoes and other veggies grown from heirloom seeds, you would want to have these even if our access to unaltered seeds were not imperiled.

While some nations have banned genetically altered foods, and others are fighting to keep these foods from their borders, here in the U.S. very few Americans know anything about the issue. Some estimates place the ratio of food on our grocery shelves containing genetically engineered organisms at 60 to 70 percent. The biotech industry intends to genetically engineer all of the food in the world within 5 or 10 years. These foods are not subjected to proper long-term safety testing before they hit the market, and none of them are labeled.

In 1999 most major media outlets across the nation reported that Monarch butterflies died unexpectedly from eating milkweed plants that had been dusted with pollen from genetically engineered corn containing components of the bacteria *Bacillus thuringiensis,* better known as Bt. Spliced into the DNA of corn or potatoes, Bt causes the plants to produce an insecticide naturally generated by the bacteria. Once again, this sounds promising at first, because it allows farmers to use less chemical pesticide, and because Bt breaks down rapidly in the ground and affects only the target pests. But organic farmers also use Bt in spray form to control beetle infestations on potatoes, for example. With huge amounts of Bt being engineered into potatoes by one major corporation, it seems inevitable that potato beetles and other pests will develop resistance to it, and when that happens, organic farmers will lose a relatively harmless natural pesticide.

Genetic engineering can create unexpected and hard-to-detect toxins and allergens and can reduce the nutritional value of our foods. The British Medical Association is calling for a moratorium on transgenic plantings. In April 1999, the seven largest grocery chains in six European countries made a public commitment to go "GE free"–to eliminate genetically engineered ingredients from their products and stores. Over 1,300 schools in the United Kingdom have banned these foods from their cafeterias. The European Union is demanding segregation and labeling of all GE imports. Even the Pope has warned of the ethical implications of genetic engineering of food!

Another practice that threatens to distort the way agriculture is practiced on a worldwide basis is known as monoculture, which David M. Soderquist has defined as "the destruction of a diverse ecosystem and replacement with a single species system. This is most often a crop of little local value, but with enormous direct and/or indirect profit potentials in other regions or countries." Typical examples include the conversion of Latin American or East Asian economies to produce mainly bananas, rubber, or sugar cane for export to the U.S. Through various tax incentives to the large corporations creating monocultures abroad, American taxpayers ultimately subsidize the construction of roads and airstrips to facilitate export of these products.

You can express your concern about genetic engineering and monoculture to, and demand responses from, the following governmental agencies:

Daniel Glickman, Secretary, USDA, 14 Independence Ave. SW, Washington, DC 20250 (202 720-3631), agsec@usda.gov

FDA Consumer Protection Agency, 5600 Fishers La, Rockville, MD 20857 (888 463-6332), www.fda.gov

National Institutes of Health, Bethesda, MD 20892 (301 496-4000)

ORGANIC HEIRLOOM SEEDS SUPPLIERS

The Cooks Garden
Box 535
Londonderry, VT 05148

Johnny's Selected Seeds
1 Foss Hill Rd.
RR 1 Box 2580
Albion, ME 04910-9731

Seed of Change
Box 15700
Sante Fe, NM 87506-5700

Seeds Blum Heirloom Seeds
HC 33 Idaho City Stage
Boise, ID 83706

Shepards Garden Seeds
30 Irene St.
Torrington, CT 06790
(800) 444-6910

Southern Exposure
Box 170
Earlyville, VA 22936

PRIVATE ORGANIC CERTIFICATION ORGANIZATIONS

Appalachian Mushroom Growers Association
RR 1, Box 30BYY
Haywood, VA 22722
(703) 923-4774
Contact: John Lombardi
Region of Operation: Virginia

California Certified Organic Farmers (CCOF)
State Office
1115 Mission St.
Santa Cruz, CA 95060
(408) 423-2263; fax (408) 423-4528

Contact: Diane Bowen, Executive Director
Region of Operation: California and other states whose home office is in California

Carolina Farm Stewardship Association (CFSA)
Box 448
Pittsboro, NC 27312
(919) 542-2402; fax (919) 542-7401
cfsa@sunsite.unc.edu
Contact: Laura Lauffer
Region of Operation: North Carolina, South Carolina

The Demeter Association, Inc.
Britt Rd.
Aurora, NY 13026
(315) 364-5617; fax (315) 364-5224
Contact: Anne Mendenhall
Region of Operation: International

Farm Verified Organic, Inc. (FVO)
5449 45 St. SE
Medina, ND 58467
(701) 486-3578; fax (701) 486-3580
farmvo@daktel.com
Contact: Annie Kirschenmann, Program Manager
Region of Operation: International

Florida Organic Growers & Consumers, Inc. (FOGC)
Box 12311
Gainesville, FL 32604
(352) 377-6345; fax (352) 377-8363
fogoffice@aol.com
Contact: Marty Mesh
Region of Operation: International

Georgia Organic Growers Association (GOGA)
4400 Happy Valley Circle
Newnan, GA 30263
(770) 253-0347; fax (770) 253-0347
GOGAcertif@aol.com
Contact: Larry Conklin, Certification Coordinator
Region of Operation: Georgia, Alabama

Global Organic Alliance
Box 530
Bellofante, OH 43311-0530
(937) 593-1232
Contact: Betty Kananen

Hawaii Bioorganic Growers Association (HBGA)
Box 800
Honaunau (Kona), HI 96726
(808) 328-2083; fax (808) 328-9760
Contact: Robert Faust, Managing Officer
Region of Operation: Hawaii

Hawaii Organic Farmers Association (HOFA)
431 Lilikoi Rd.
Haiku (Maui), HI 96708
(808) 573-0995; fax (808) 573-0995
hofa@aloha.net
Contact: Diana Dahl
Region of Operation: Hawaii

Indiana Certified Organic
1168 N CR 575 W
Greencastle, IN 46135
(765) 653-8933)
Vcarr@ccrtc.com

Contact: Val Carr
Region of Operation: Indiana and surrounding states

Kauai Organic Growers Association (KOGA)
4480 Omao Rd.
Koloa (Kauai), HI 96756
(808) 742-1479
Contact: Phil Sheldon, President
Region of Operation: Hawaii (Kauai only)

Living Farms, Inc.
Box 50
Tracy, MN 56175
(507) 629-4431; fax (507) 629-4253
Contact: Ardell Anderson
Region of Operation: Midwest

Maine Organic Farmers & Gardeners Association (MOFGA)
Box 2176
Augusta, ME 04338-2176
(207) 622-3118; fax (207) 622-3119
mofga@biddeford.com
Contact: Russell Libby
Region of Operation: Maine

Mountain State Organic Growers & Buyers Association (MSOGBA)
1145 Back Valley Rd.
Sweet Spring, WV 24941
(703) 897-5741
Contact: Vivian Purdy
Region of Operation: West Virginia

Northeast Organic Farming Association Connecticut (NOFACT)
Box 386

Northford, CT 06472-0386
Contact: Melvin Lee Bristol, Certification Committee Cochair
Region of Operation: Connecticut

Northeast Organic Farming Association Massachusetts (NOFAMA)
140 Chestnut St.
West Hatfield, MA 01088
(413) 247-9264
Contact: Edwin McGlew, Administrator
Region of Operation: Massachusetts

Northeast Organic Farming Association New Jersey (NOFANJ)
33 Titus Mill Rd.
Bennington, NJ 08534
(609) 737-6848; fax (609) 737-2366
nofanj@aol.com
Contact: Karen Anderson
Region of Operation: New Jersey, Pennsylvania

Northeast Organic Farming Association New York (NOFANY)
26 Towpath Rd.
Binghamton, NY 13904
(607) 724-9853; fax (607) 648-8640
Contact: Patricia Kane, Administrator
Region of Operation: New York, Pennsylvania

Northeast Organic Farming Association Vermont (NOFAVT)
Box 697
Richmond, VT 05477
fax (802) 434-4154
Contact: Enid Wonnacott, Certification Administrator
Region of Operation: Vermont, New York, Pennsylvania

Ohio Ecological Food & Farming Association (OEFFA)
Box 82234
Columbus, OH 43202

(614) 294-3663; fax (614) 291-3276
oeffa@iwaynet.net
Contact: Sylvia Upp, Certification Coordinator
Region of Operation: Ohio, Pennsylvania, Kentucky, Indiana, and nearby states

Oregon Tilth Certified Organically Grown (OTCOG)
1860 Hawthorne Ave. NE
Suite 200
Salem, OR 97303
(503) 378-0690; fax (503) 378-0809
organic@tilth.org
Contact: Yvonne Frost, Executive Director
Region of Operation: International

Organic Certification Services, Inc. (OCS)
128 Mason Rd.
Melrose, FL 32666
(352) 475-2037
Contact: Robin Lauriault, President
Region of Operation: Florida

Organic Crop Improvement Association (OCIA)
1101 Y St.
Suite B
Lincoln, NE 68508-1172
(402) 477-2323; fax (402) 477-4325
www.ocia.org
Contact: Krista Kennedy
Region of Operation: International

Organic Forum International
514 Lynne Ave.
Ypsilanti, MI 48198-4262
(313) 480-4262
organicforum@ameritech.net

Contact: Mike Pratt
Region of Operation: International

Organic Growers & Buyers Association (OGBA)
1405 Silver Lake Rd.
New Brighton, MN 55112
(612) 572-1967; fax 612 572-2527
Contact: Sue Cristan
Region of Operation: International

Organic Growers of Michigan
135 E. 120 St.
Grant, MI 49327
(616) 834-5481
Contact: Gray Larison
Region of Operation: Michigan

Organic Verification Organization of North America (OVONA) U.S.
Box 146
Hitterdale, MN 56552
(218) 962-3264; fax (218) 962-3264
Contact: Matthew Moe
Region of Operation: National (with Canadian affiliate)

Pennsylvania Certified Organic
Box 452
Centre Hall, PA
(814) 364-1344
Contact: Tom Beddard
Region of Operation: Pennsylvania

Quality Assurance International (QAI)
12526 High Bluff Dr.
Suite 300
San Diego, CA 92130
(619) 792-3531; fax (619) 755-8665

Contact: Griffith W. McLellan, Director
East Coast Office
150 Dorset St. #246
South Burlington, VT 05407
(819) 877-2663
Contact: Joe Smillie
Region of Operation: International

Scientific Certification Systems (SCS)
(Nutriclean Organic Certification Program)
1939 Harrison St.
Suite 400
Oakland, CA 94612
(510) 832-1415; fax (510) 832-0359
Contact: Zoe Kilkenny, Operations Manager
Region of Operation: National

Tennessee Land Stewardship Association (TLSA)
450 Davidson Chapel Lane
Bloomington Springs, TN 38545
(931) 653-4402; fax (931) 653-4545
bshine@infoave.net
Contact: Bob Shine, Coordinator
Region of Operation: Tennessee

Tidewater Organic Growers Association (TOGA)
RR 640, Box 3360
Water View, VA 23180
Contact: Iris Fellers
Region of Operation: Virginia

United States Assurance Laboratories (USAL)
4150 Colfax Ave. North
Minneapolis, MN 55412
(612) 522-8224; fax (612) 228-9937

Contact: Luddene E. Perry, Managing Director
Region of Operation: National

Vermont Maple Sugarmaker's Association, Inc. (VMSA)
RR 1, Box 3500
Westford, VT 05494
Contact: Sandra Tarrier, Secretary
Region of Operation: Vermont

Virginia Biological Farmers Association (VABF)
RR 1, Box 46
Check, VA 24072
(540) 651-4747
Contact: Donna Whitmarsh, Certification Coordinator
Region of Operation: Virginia

Appendix 3

SPRING GROCERY SHOPPING LIST

GENERAL GUIDELINES

- In summer, eat off the summer list.
- In winter, eat off the winter list.
- In spring, eat off the spring list.
- Think in terms of increasing good foods in season rather than avoiding foods.
- Remember, there are no bad foods—if your favorite food does not appear in one season, wait a couple of months and it will show up on the next season's list.
- In spring, eat a low-fat diet taking more salads, veggies, leafy greens, beans, sprouts, and berries.
- In summer, eat more fruits and veggies, as they are almost pure carbohydrates.
- In winter, eat more nuts, grains, soups, and meats to ensure the storage of protein and fats for the winter.
- Read chapter 7 to tailor the 3-Season Diet to your body type and geographic location.
- See the Glossary of Foods (Appendix 1) for details on common foods.

KEY

1. Best   Best season for this food
2. Good   Second-best season for this food
3. Reduce   Eat small amounts, if any
4. Avoid   Try to eliminate this food

SPRING

FRUIT		REDUCE	AVOID
Apples	Good	Apricots	Figs
Blueberries	Good	Bananas	Guava

291

SPRING

FRUIT			REDUCE	AVOID
Dried Fruits	Best		Cantaloupe	
Grapefruit	Good		Cherries	
Lemons	Good		Coconuts	
Limes	Good		Cranberries	
Papayas	Good		Dates	
Pears	Good		Grapes	
Pomegranates	Good		Mangoes	
Raspberries	Good		Melons	
Strawberries	Good		Nectarines	
			Oranges	
			Peaches	
			Persimmons	
			Pineapples	
			Plums	
			Tangerines	

VEGETABLES			REDUCE	AVOID
Alfalfa Sprouts	Best		Avocados	
Artichokes	Good		Cucumbers	
Asparagus	Best		Eggplant	
Bean Sprouts	Best		Okra	
Beets	Good		Squash, Acorn	
Bell Peppers	Best		Squash, Winter	
Bitter Melon	Good		Sweet Potatoes	
Broccoli	Good		Pumpkins	
Brussels Sprouts	Best		Tomatoes	
Cabbage	Best		Zucchini, unless cooked	
Carrots	Best			
Cauliflower	Best			
Celery	Best			
Chicory	Best			

SPRING

VEGETABLES		REDUCE	AVOID
Chilies	Best, dried		
Cilantro	Good		
Collard Greens	Best		
Corn	Best		
Dandelions	Best		
Endive	Best		
Fennel	Good		
Garlic	Best		
Ginger	Good		
Green Beans	Best		
Hot Peppers	Best		
Jicama	Good		
Kale	Best		
Leeks	Good		
Lettuce	Best		
Mushrooms	Best		
Mustard Greens	Best		
Onions	Best		
Parsley	Best		
Peas	Best		
Peas, Snow	Good		
Potatoes	Good, baked		
Seaweed	Good		
Spinach	Best		
Swiss Chard	Best		
Radishes	Best		
Turnips	Best		
Watercress	Best		

GRAINS		REDUCE	AVOID
Amaranth	Good	Wheat	
Barley	Good	Rice	

SPRING

GRAINS		REDUCE	AVOID
Buckwheat	Good		
Corn	Good		
Millet	Good		
Oats	Good, dry		
Quinoa	Good		
Rice, Brown	Good, long grain		
Rye	Good		

LEGUMES		REDUCE	AVOID
Bean Sprouts	Best	Tofu	
Adzukis	Good		
Black Grams	Good		
Garbanzos	Good		
Favas	Good		
Goyas	Best		
Kidneys	Best		
Lentils	Best		
Limas	Best		
Mungs	Best		
Split Peas	Good		

NUTS/SEEDS		REDUCE	AVOID
Filberts	Good	Coconuts	Almonds
Piñons	Good		Brazil Nuts
Pumpkin	Good		Cashews
Sunflower	Good		Flax
			Lotus Seed
			Macadamias
			Peanuts, raw
			Pecans
			Pistachios
			Walnuts

SPRING

DAIRY		REDUCE	AVOID
Ghee	Good in moderation	Butter, eat before sunset	Ice Cream
Low Fat Yogurt	Good in moderation	Buttermilk	
Rice/Soy Milk	Good	Cheese	
		Cottage Cheese	
		Cream	
		Kefir	
		Milk, low fat or skim	
		Sour Cream	

MEAT AND FISH		REDUCE	AVOID
Chicken	Good	Beef	Crabs
Duck	Good in moderation	Oysters	Lobster
Eggs	Good in moderation	Shrimp	Pork
Freshwater Fish	Good	Venison	
Lamb	Good in moderation		
Ocean Fish	Good in moderation		
Turkey	Good		

OILS		REDUCE	AVOID
In general: All oils in moderation			
Canola	Good	Almond	Peanut
Corn	Best	Avocado	
Flax	Good	Coconut	
Mustard	Good	Olive	
Safflower	Good	Sesame	

SPRING

OILS		REDUCE	AVOID
Soy	Good		
Sunflower	Good		

SWEETENERS		REDUCE	AVOID
Honey	Best	Raw Sugar	
Maple syrup	Good	Rice Syrup	
Molasses	Good	White Sugar	

CONDIMENTS		REDUCE	AVOID
Carob	Good	Mayonnaise	
Chocolate	Good, reduce	Salt	
Pickles	Good	Vinegar	

BEVERAGES		REDUCE	AVOID
Black Tea	Good	Alcohol	
Coffee	Good		
Sparkling Water	Good		

HERB TEAS			
Alfalfa	Good		
Cardamom	Best		
Chamomile	Reduce		
Chicory	Best		
Cinnamon	Best		
Cloves	Best		
Dandelion	Best		
Ginger	Best		
Hibiscus	Best		
Mint	Reduce		

SPRING

HERB TEAS			
Orange Peel	Best		
Strawberry Leaf	Best		

SPICES		REDUCE	AVOID
Anise	Good		
Asafoetida	Good		
Basil	Good		
Bay Leaf	Good		
Black Pepper	Best		
Chamomile	Good		
Caraway	Good		
Cardamom	Good		
Cayenne	Best		
Cinnamon	Good		
Clove	Best		
Coriander	Good		
Cumin	Good		
Dill	Good		
Fennel	Good		
Fenugreek	Good		
Garlic	Good		
Ginger	Good		
Horseradish	Good		
Marjoram	Good		
Mustard	Good		
Nutmeg	Good		
Oregano	Good		
Peppermint	Good		
Poppy Seeds	Good		
Rosemary	Good		
Saffron	Good		
Sage	Good		

SPRING

SPICES		REDUCE	AVOID
Spearmint	Good		
Thyme	Good		
Turmeric	Good		

SUMMER GROCERY SHOPPING LIST

GENERAL GUIDELINES

- In summer, eat off the summer list.
- In winter, eat off the winter list.
- In spring, eat off the spring list.
- Think in terms of increasing good foods in season rather than avoiding foods.
- Remember, there are no bad foods–if your favorite food does not appear in one season, wait a couple of months and it will show up on the next season's list.
- In spring, eat a low-fat diet by taking more salads, veggies, leafy greens, beans, sprouts, and berries.
- In summer, eat more fruits and veggies, as they are almost pure carbohydrates.
- In winter, eat more nuts, grains, soups, and meats to ensure the storage of protein and fats for the winter.
- Read chapter 7 to tailor the 3-Season Diet to your body type and geographic location.
- See the Glossary of Foods, (Appendix 1) for details on common foods.

KEY

1. Best — Best season for this food
2. Good — Second-best season for this food
3. Reduce — Eat small amounts, if any
4. Avoid — Try to eliminate this food

SUMMER

FRUIT		REDUCE	AVOID
Apples	Best	Grapefruit	
Apricots	Best	Lemons	
Bananas	Good	Limes	
Blueberries	Best	Sour Fruits	
Cantaloupe	Best		

SUMMER

FRUIT		REDUCE	AVOID
Cherries	Best, ripe		
Coconuts	Best, green or ripe		
Cranberries	Best		
Dates	Good		
Dried Fruit	Good		
Figs	Good		
Grapes	Best		
Guava	Best		
Mangoes	Best		
Melons	Best		
Nectarines	Good		
Oranges	Good, sweet		
Papayas	Good, sm. amts.		
Peaches	Good, tree ripe		
Pears	Best		
Persimmons	Best		
Pineapples	Best, sweet		
Plums	Best, ripe		
Pomegranates	Best		
Raspberries	Best		
Strawberries	Best		
Tangerines	Good, sweet		

VEGETABLES		REDUCE	AVOID
Alfalfa Sprouts	Good	Carrots	Beets
Artichokes	Best	Garlic	Brussels Sprouts
Asparagus	Best	Ginger	
Avocados	Good	Hot Peppers	
Bean Sprouts	Good	Leeks	
Beet Greens	Best	Onions, unless cooked	
Bell Peppers	Best	Radishes	

SUMMER

VEGETABLES		REDUCE	AVOID
Bitter Melon	Best	Turnips	
Broccoli	Best		
Cabbage	Best		
Cauliflower	Best		
Celery	Best		
Chicory	Good		
Cilantro	Best		
Collard Greens	Good		
Corn	Good		
Cucumbers	Best		
Dandelions	Best		
Endive	Good		
Fennel	Best		
Eggplant	Good		
Green Beans	Good		
Jicama	Best		
Kale	Best		
Lettuce	Best		
Mushrooms	Good		
Mustard Greens	Good		
Okra	Best		
Parsley	Good		
Peas	Good		
Peas, Snow	Best		
Pumpkin	Good		
Seaweed	Good		
Spinach	Good in moderation		
Squash, Acorn	Best		
Squash, Winter	Good		
Sweet Potatoes	Good		
Swiss Chard	Good		

SUMMER

VEGETABLES		REDUCE	AVOID
Tomatoes	Good, vine ripe & sweet in moderation		
Turnip Greens	Good		
Watercress	Best		
Zucchini	Best		

GRAINS		REDUCE	AVOID
Barley	Best	Amaranth	
Rye	Good	Buckwheat	
Wheat	Good	Corn	
Oat	Good	Millet	
Rice	Best	Quinoa	
		Rice, Brown	

LEGUMES		REDUCE	AVOID
Adzukis	Best		
Bean Sprouts	Good		
Black Grams	Best		
Favas	Best		
Garbanzos	Best		
Goyas	Good		
Kidneys	Good		
Lentils	Good		
Limas	Good		
Mungs	Good		
Split Pea	Best		
Tofu	Best		

NUTS/SEEDS		REDUCE	AVOID
Almonds	Good	Brazil Nuts	
Coconut	Best	Cashews	

SUMMER

NUTS/SEEDS		REDUCE	AVOID
Flax	Good	Peanuts, raw	
Macadamias	Good	Filberts	
Piñon	Good	Pecans	
Pumpkin	Best	Pistachios	
Sunflower	Best	Walnuts	

DAIRY		REDUCE	AVOID
Butter	Good	Buttermilk	
Cheese	Good in moderation	Kefir	
Cottage Cheese	Good	Sour Cream	
		Yogurt	
Ghee	Best		
Ice Cream	Good		
Milk	Best		
Rice/Soy Milk	Best		

MEAT AND FISH		REDUCE	AVOID
Beef	Good in moderation	Venison	
Chicken	Good	Lobster	
Duck	Good in moderation	Oysters	
Eggs	Good in moderation	Crabs	
Freshwater Fish	Good		
Lamb	Good in moderation		
Pork	Good		
Shrimp	Good in moderation		
Turkey	Good		

SUMMER

OILS		REDUCE	AVOID
Almond	Good	Corn	
Avocado	Good	Mustard	
Canola	Good	Peanut	
Coconut	Best	Safflower	
Flax	Good	Sesame	
Olive	Best		
Soy	Best		
Sunflower	Good		

SWEETENERS		REDUCE	AVOID
Maple Syrup	Good	Honey	
Raw Sugar	Good	Molasses	
Rice Syrup	Good	White Sugar	

CONDIMENTS		REDUCE	AVOID
Carob	Good	Chocolate	
Mayonnaise	Good	Pickles	
		Salt	
		Vinegar	

BEVERAGES		REDUCE	AVOID
Sparkling Water	Good or reduce (depending on body type)	Alcohol	
		Black Tea	

HERB TEAS		REDUCE	AVOID
Alfalfa	Good		
Cardamom	Reduce		
Chamomile	Best		

SUMMER

HERB TEAS		REDUCE	AVOID
Chicory	Best		
Cinnamon	Reduce		
Cloves	Reduce		
Dandelion	Best		
Ginger	Reduce		
Hibiscus	Best		
Mint	Best		
Orange Peel	Reduce		
Strawberry Leaf	Reduce		

SPICES		REDUCE	AVOID
Anise	Good		
Asafoetida	Good		
Basil	Reduce		
Bay Leaf	Reduce		
Black Pepper	Reduce		
Chamomile	Best		
Caraway	Reduce		
Cardamom	Reduce		
Cayenne	Reduce		
Cinnamon	Reduce		
Clove	Reduce		
Coriander	Best		
Cumin	Good		
Dill	Reduce		
Fennel	Good		
Fenugreek	Reduce		
Garlic	Reduce		
Ginger	Reduce		
Horseradish	Reduce		
Marjoram	Reduce		
Mustard	Reduce		

SUMMER

SPICES		REDUCE	AVOID
Nutmeg	Good or Reduce (depending on body type)		
Oregano	Reduce		
Peppermint	Good		
Poppy Seeds	Reduce		
Rosemary	Good or Reduce (depending on body type)		
Saffron	Good		
Sage	Reduce		
Spearmint	Good		
Thyme	Reduce		
Turmeric	Good		

WINTER GROCERY SHOPPING LIST

GENERAL GUIDELINES

- In summer, eat off the summer list.
- In winter, eat off the winter list.
- In spring, eat off the spring list.
- Think in terms of increasing good foods in season rather than avoiding foods.
- Remember, there are no bad foods—if your favorite food does not appear in one season, wait a couple of months and it will show up on the next season's list.
- In spring, eat a low-fat diet by taking more salads, veggies, leafy greens, beans, sprouts, and berries.
- In summer, eat more fruits and veggies, as they are almost pure carbohydrates.
- In winter, eat more nuts, grains, soups, and meats to ensure the storage of protein and fats for the winter.
- Read chapter 7 to tailor the 3-Season Diet to your body type and geographic location.
- See the Glossary of Foods (Appendix 1) for details on common foods.

KEY

1. Best — Best season for this food
2. Good — Second-best season for this food
3. Reduce — Eat small amounts, if any
4. Avoid — Try to eliminate this food

WINTER

FRUIT		REDUCE	AVOID
Apples	Good, cooked		
Apricots	Good	Apples, raw	
Bananas	Best	Fresh Cranberries	
Blueberries	Good	Melons	
Cantaloupe	Good w/lemon	Pomegranates	

WINTER

FRUIT		REDUCE	AVOID
Cherries	Good	Raspberries	
Coconuts	Good, ripe		
Cranberries	Good, cooked	Unripe Fruit	
Dates	Best		
Figs	Best		
Grapefruit	Best		
Grapes	Best		
Guava	Good		
Lemons	Best		
Limes	Best		
Mangoes	Best		
Nectarines	Good		
Oranges	Best		
Papayas	Best		
Peaches	Good		
Pears	Good, ripe		
Persimmons	Best		
Pineapples	Good		
Plums	Good		
Strawberries	Good		
Tangerines	Best		

VEGETABLES		REDUCE	AVOID
Artichokes	Good, hearts	Alfalfa Sprouts	Bean Sprouts
Avocados	Best	Asparagus	Cabbage
Beets	Best	Bell Peppers, unless cooked	Cauliflower
Brussels Sprouts	Best	Broccoli, unless cooked	Cilantro
Carrots	Best	Celery, unless cooked	Collard Greens
Chilies	Best	Chicory	Cucumbers

WINTER

VEGETABLES		REDUCE	AVOID
Corn	Good	Endive	Dandelions
Fennel	Good	Green Beans, unless cooked	
Eggplant	Good, if cooked	Hibiscus	
Garlic	Best	Jicama, unless cooked	
Ginger	Good	Kale, unless cooked	
Hot Peppers	Good	Lettuce	
Leeks	Good	Mushrooms	
Okra	Good	Mustard Greens, unless cooked	
Onions	Good	Peas, unless cooked	
Parsley	Good	Peas, Snow	
Potatoes	Good, mashed	Radishes	
Pumpkins	Best	Spinach	
Seaweed	Good, cooked	Swiss Chard	
Squash, Acorn	Good	Watercress	
Squash, Winter	Best	Zucchini, unless cooked	
Sweet Potatoes	Best		
Tomatoes	Best		
Turnips	Good		

GRAINS		REDUCE	AVOID
Amaranth	Best	Barley	
Buckwheat	Good in moderation	Corn, okay in moderation	
Millet	Good in moderation	Oats, dry	
Oats	Best		
Quinoa	Best		

WINTER

GRAINS		REDUCE	AVOID
Rice	Good		
Rice, Brown	Best		
Rye	Good in moderation		
Wheat	Best		

LEGUMES		REDUCE	AVOID
Mungs		Adzukis	
Tofu		Bean Sprouts	
		Black Grams	
		Favas	
		Garbanzos	
		Goyas	
		Kidneys	
		Lentils	
		Limas	
		Split Peas	

NUTS/SEEDS		REDUCE	AVOID
Almonds	Best	Pumpkin	
Brazil Nuts	Best		
Cashews	Best		
Coconuts	Good		
Filberts	Best		
Flax	Best		
Lotus Seed	Good		
Macadamias	Best		
Peanuts, raw	Best		
Pecans	Best		
Piñons	Best		
Pistachios	Best		

WINTER

NUTS/SEEDS		REDUCE	AVOID
Sunflower	Good		
Walnuts	Best		

DAIRY		REDUCE	AVOID
Butter	Best		Ice Cream
Buttermilk	Best		
Cheese	Best		
Cottage Cheese	Best		
Cream	Best		
Ghee	Best		
Kefir	Best		
Milk	Good, not cold		
Rice/Soy Milk	Good		
Sour Cream	Good		
Yogurt	Good		

MEAT AND FISH		REDUCE	AVOID
Beef	Best		
Chicken	Best		
Crabs	Best		
Duck	Best		
Eggs	Best		
Freshwater fish	Best		
Lamb	Best		
Lobster	Best		
Ocean Fish	Best		
Oysters	Best		
Pork	Best		
Shrimp	Best		
Turkey	Best		
Venison	Best		

WINTER

OILS		REDUCE	AVOID
Almond	Best		
Avocado	Best		
Canola	Best		
Coconut	Best		
Corn	Good		
Flax	Best		
Mustard	Best		
Olive	Best		
Peanut	Best		
Safflower	Best		
Sesame	Best		
Soy	Good		
Sunflower	Good		

SWEETENERS		REDUCE	AVOID
Honey	Good	White Sugar	
Maple Syrup	Best		
Molasses	Best		
Raw Sugar	Good		
Rice Syrup	Best		

CONDIMENTS		REDUCE	AVOID
Carob	Good		
Chocolate	Good		
Mayonnaise	Good		
Pickles	Good		
Salt	Best		
Vinegar	Good		

WINTER

BEVERAGES			REDUCE	AVOID
Alcohol	(moderation)			
Alcohol	Good			
Black Tea				
Coffee				
Sparkling Water				

HERB TEAS			REDUCE	AVOID
Cardamom	Best		Alfalfa	
Chamomile	Best		Chicory	
Cinnamon	Best		Dandelion	
Cloves	Best		Hibiscus	
Ginger	Best		Strawberry Leaf	
Mint	Good			
Orange Peel	Best			

SPICES			REDUCE	AVOID
Anise	Best			
Asafoetida	Best			
Basil	Best			
Bay Leaf	Good			
Black Pepper	Best			
Caraway	Good			
Cardamom	Best			
Cayenne	Good			
Chamomile	Good			
Cinnamon	Best			
Clove	Good			
Coriander	Good			
Cumin	Best			
Dill	Good			
Fennel	Best			

WINTER

SPICES		REDUCE	AVOID
Fenugreek	Good		
Garlic	Good		
Ginger	Best		
Horseradish	Good		
Marjoram	Good		
Mustard	Good		
Nutmeg	Good		
Oregano	Good		
Peppermint	Good		
Poppy Seeds	Good		
Rosemary	Good		
Saffron	Best		
Sage	Good		
Spearmint	Good		
Thyme	Good		
Turmeric	Best		

Bibliography

Atkins, Robert C., M.D. *Dr. Atkins' Health Revolution.* New York: Bantam, 1998.

DesMaisons, Katherine, Ph.D. *Potatoes Not Prozac.* New York: Fireside, 1999.

Diamond, Harvey and Marilyn. *Fit for Life.* New York: Warner Books, 1985.

Douillard, John. *Body, Mind and Sport.* New York: Harmony, 1994.

Erasmus, U. *Fats and Oils.* Burnaby, B.C., Canada: Alive Books, 1987.

Frawley, David. *American Institute of Vedic Studies—Course Material Part 4.* Santa Fe, N.M.: A.I.V.S. [no date]

Haas, Elson M., M.D. *A Diet for All Seasons.* Berkeley: Celestial Arts, 1995.

Haas, Robert. *Eat To Win.* New York: Rawson Associates, 1983.

Jensen, Dr. Bernard. *Nature Has a Remedy: A Book of Remedies for Body, Mind, and Spirit Gathered from All Corners of the World.* Escondido, Ca., 1978.

——— *Foods That Heal: A Guide to Understanding and Using the Healing Powers of Natural Foods.* Garden City Park, N.Y.: Avery Publishing Group, 1988.

Kapoor, L.D. *CRC Handbook of Ayurvedic Medicinal Plants.* Boca Raton, Fla.: CRC Press, 1990.

Krause, M. and K. Mahan, *Food, Nutrition and Diet Therapy.* Philadelphia, Pa.: W. B. Saunders Co., 1979.

Kreutler, Patricia A. *Nutrition in Perspective.* Englewood Cliffs, N.J.: Prentice-Hall, 1980.

McDougall, John A. and Mary A. *The McDougall Plan.* Piscataway, N.J.: New Century Publishers, 1983.

Pritikin, Nathan. *Diet for Runners.* New York: Simon & Schuster, 1985.

Sada Shiva Tirtha, S. *The Ayurveda Encyclopedia.* Bayville, N.Y.: Ayurveda Holistic Center Press, 1998.

Sears, Barry, Ph.D., *The Zone.* New York: HarperCollins, 1995.

Sheldon, William H., Ph.D., M.D. *Atlas of Men: A Guide for Somatotyping the Adult Male at All Ages.* New York: Gramercy Publishing, 1954.

Steward, H. Leighton, et al. *Sugar Busters!* New York: Ballantine, 1998.

Tiwari, Bri. Maya. *A Life in Balance.* Rochester, Vt.: Healing Arts Press, 1995.

ARTICLES

Brody, Jane E. "New Look at Dieting: Fat Can Be a Friend." *The New York Times,* May 25, 1999, p. F1.

——— "Doubts Fail to Deter 'The Diet Revolution.'" *The New York Times,* May 25, 1999, p. F7.

Loomis, Susan Herrmann. "Paradox? What Paradox? The French Are Finally Getting Fat." *The New York Times,* Sept. 9, 1998.

Winckler, Suzanne. "A Savage Life." *The New York Times Magazine,* Feb. 7, 1999.

Zafar, R., and S. M. Ali. "Anti-Hepatotoxic Effects of Root and Root-Callus Extracts of *Cichorium intybus L.*" *Journal of Ethnopharmacology,* 1998, 63:227–331.

Index

Achieve personal peak performance levels
with John Douillard's "gain without pain"
approach to physical fitness.

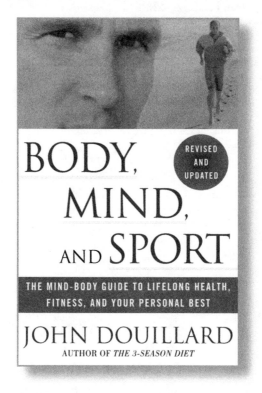

BODY, MIND, AND SPORT
The Mind-Body Guide to Lifelong Health,
Fitness, and Your Personal Best

"I have been on John Douillard's program for eight months now
and never have I felt better. ... Everything about me is balanced—
the emotional, mental, and physical are working in balance."
—From the Foreword by Martina Navratilova

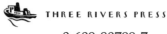 THREE RIVERS PRESS

0-609-80789-7
$14.00 paper (Canada: $21.00)
AVAILABLE WHEREVER BOOKS ARE SOLD